Journeys
of
Grief *and* Loss

....

DR. MAPLE MELDER CROZIER

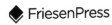 FriesenPress

One Printers Way
Altona, MB R0G0B0
Canada

www.friesenpress.com

ISBN
978-1-03-910232-3 (Hardcover)
978-1-03-910231-6 (Paperback)
978-1-03-910233-0 (eBook)

1. Self-Help, Death, Grief, Bereavement

Distributed to the trade by The Ingram Book Company

Table of Contents

"No one's getting out of this world alive."

Anonymous

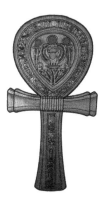

Introduction

"Grief is the price we pay for love."
Queen Elizabeth II

INTRODUCTION

The fabric of humanity is knit together by the certainty, the commonality, the reality of several things; the most elemental of these things being that we will all die. There are few other absolute truths. Benjamin Franklin (n.d.) is credited with positing that "Nothing can be said to be certain, except death and taxes." Some people have avoided the taxes. Death, however, looms for us all.

Did the bluntness of the statement surprise you? In progressive, developed cultures of much of the United States and Canada, we often do not discuss death. Grief counselling specialist Dr. Alan Wolfelt declares, "We live in a grief-avoidant culture" (2016). Death, and the concomitant grief, is a shadowy experience, dressed in black and spoken of in hushed terms. It is treated somberly and seriously, exemplified by the lived experience at most funerals. Though some people add cultural and religious rituals, it is generally experienced as crying at a funeral or memorial service, and then moving on.

Do we really move on? Death brings a disconnect between head and heart. You know the person is gone, but your heart doesn't want to let go of them. You have heard the details from the doctor or the police, but it just doesn't make sense. You can't reconcile the news with yesterday's reality of life. It's this push and pull, this tug-of-war that takes such energy and sleep from us.

With death comes grief. Most research suggests we move through grief (Wolfelt, 2016), not on from it. There is no set pace or timeline. There is no one pathway. There is no one right way to grieve. There is no standard for how to live out this experience. Jamie Anderson (n.d.) said, "Grief, I've learned, is really just love. It's all the love you want to give, but cannot. All that unspent love gathers up in the corners of your eyes, the lump in your throat, and in that hollow part of your chest. Grief is just love with no place to go."

Everyone experiences loss. It could be loss of a home, a best friend, or a school because of moving. It could be the loss of a pet. It could be a miscarriage or an abortion, or the discovery of infertility, or the challenge of giving a child up for adoption. It could be the death of a parent or sibling, a friend or partner. Another significant loss is the loss of safety and security because of trauma.

Loss comes in many forms. And with loss there is grief.

That is the reason for this book. In this volume I will present the journey of grief and loss from the perspectives of eleven individuals. This journey will be shared through their words and through pictures of the memorials they and others have created to remember their loved ones. In her book *When You Lose Someone You Love,* Joanne Fink (2019) shares, "I've discovered that grieving is like taking a journey toward an unknown destination against your will: it is incredibly difficult, heartbreaking, and time consuming—and there aren't any shortcuts."

Because of that reality, this book will discuss many of the certainties of death. It will also consider the uncertainties of life for the survivors after the death of a loved one, that the eleven people interviewed have experienced.

If you have lost a loved one, you'll be able to relate to the stories shared here. If you haven't lost someone or something very precious to you, you will. It is the natural order of life to include death. As Fink (2019) continued, "Most of us will experience the loss of someone we love and need to deal with that loss in order to move on with our life's journey."

It is for the living that we learn about grief and loss. In fact, research shows 15 percent of all psychological disorders have unresolved grief as their source (Samuel, 2018). This confirms that the study of grief has implications in most people's lives. The stories of brave individuals in this book can be a guide for you in future journeys.

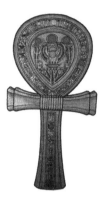

Dedication

"Love is worth it. It is always worth it.
In fact, it's the only thing that's worth anything."
Alan Wolfert, author and grief specialist

DEDICATION

I was blessed to live a great love story for over forty years with my beloved

Michael Joseph Crozier

who died April 18, 2018. Losing his love brought me a hurting heart, heavy shoulders, and aching tears for the loss. I gained, however, a deeper understanding of strength, generosity, humility, and kindness for and of others. I am so grateful for the life Mike and I had and the family we grew together. This book is because of him. It is dedicated to him. It is a work of my heart.

ACKNOWLEDGEMENTS

This book has been made possible by the brave souls who courageously shared their stories of the loss of a loved one, whether in a full interview or a short discussion. I appreciate each one. There were many tears shed in the retellings. Their hearts beat a little louder for having experienced the love and the loss.

Abbotsford Hospice Society hosted a grief support class that I participated in and wherein I met a wonderful bunch of grieving people. Leaders Kathy and Faye facilitated members Cathie, Cheryl, Darlene, Donna, Jessica, Pamela (PJ), and Tamy, and others who joined us for a coffee drop-in after the course ended. We all had lost a life partner, and through listening to each other in the group, we bonded, and my understanding that death affects us all differently, yet profoundly, was reinforced.

Cathie was one of these dear ones; she had lost her son, her husband, and her father, all in recent years, and lost a short battle with cancer herself. She was a huge cheerleader for me to write this book. She wanted to share in this work as she felt it imperative that children and youth get information about life and death in an objective way, before they are confronted with the emotional reality. Sadly, she left this earth before we could record her story. Thank you, Cathie, for your honest and amusing thoughts, and for sharing your love.

Finally, and importantly, this book is dedicated to the people who have most inspired me and continue to bless me with their love and care, my kids and grandkids: Marnie, Josh, Jonathan, Amanda, Cal, Malakhi, Sophia, Noah, and baby Mila. I am so glad to do life with all of you in it! I am so honoured to be your mom or nana and have you around me on this journey.

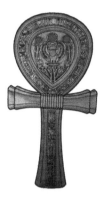

Prologue

"It takes strength to make your way through grief,
to grab hold of life and let it pull you forward."

Patti Davis, daughter of President Ronald Reagan

PURPOSE OF THIS BOOK

This book was written for those who wish to work in human service fields, specifically as child and youth care professionals. We know that all humans we work with will experience grief and loss; this is a resource for you as you support them. Disciplines who support those in loss are many, including Nursing, Social Work, and end-of-life care. This text is presented true to the Canadian Child and Youth Care (CYC) philosophy, considering positive, respectful relationships as foundational for all our lives, using a strengths-based approach to its trauma-informed practices. It is written because loss touches the lives of everyone. People involved with CYC may experience a great variety or a great number of losses in their lives, and those CYC workers working with those individuals may not have lived experience of deep loss or the death of a loved one; hence the need for this book.

Although intended for use as a text in the classroom, this book is intentionally written in a conversational style. The intimacy of the stories shared and the closeness of the discussions brought familiarity; hence this more informal format proved to be best to reflect the depth of emotions of the journeys. Though intentionally non-academic in voice, it contains many valuable resources.

The support of the Abbotsford Hospice Society (AHS) was solicited as a community partner for the writing of this book. Their vast experience in this field, and their extensive resources, were seen as invaluable to this work. The AHS was also willing to help refer persons to be interviewed for this project. As such, the Executive Director, Ron Kuehl, was contacted, and he allowed me access to Myra Lightheart, the bereavement services manager. Myra was able to contact people who had dealt with the AHS in the recent past and ask if they were interested in being interviewed. The criteria used by Myra was that the person be nineteen or older, have lost a loved one in the prior two years, and be willing to be interviewed and share their story. The names of the first people who agreed to this were then directed to me, and I set up interviews with each of them, at AHS, my office at The University of the Fraser Valley, or their home, wherever they were most comfortable. Their real names are not used in this book to maintain confidentiality.

The interviews look specifically at the loss of parents, the loss of partners, and the loss of children. No two stories are exactly alike. There are similarities and overlaps, but each brings learning. They share the diversity of experience, and commonality of feelings.

There are many losses that are not explicitly discussed in this book, including:
- loss of pets
- miscarriages
- abortions
- assisted suicide
- reactions to a group tragedy, often known as *communal grief*
- anticipatory grief as is experienced with dementia, or life-limiting diagnoses
- moving
- dreams
- innocence
- changing schools
- safety
- foster care
- adoption

Every experience of loss is unique and dependent on the history and circumstances of the people involved. The above specific areas of loss were not researched. But the experiences of loss provided in the included interviews are relatable and may give comfort.

Interviews, rather than surveys or anonymous questionnaires, were used for several reasons. Interviews are an appropriate method when there is a need to collect in-depth information on people's opinions, thoughts, experiences, and feelings. Interviews can be defined as a qualitative research technique which involves "a small number of respondents to explore their perspectives on a particular idea, program or situation" (Boyce and Neale, 2006). There are typically three different formats of interviews: structured, semi-structured, and unstructured. Semi-structured interviews were used in this research.

Individual interviews were used as a way to respect the uniqueness of individual experiences. All human service fields work from a perspective of each individual being distinctive and taking their own journey—having their own story to tell. This approach realizes that humans are complex beings with complicated lives. All their lived experiences influence who they are and how they respond to the challenges of life. The stories of loss and responses to loss that are discussed in this work are the journeys of those interviewed, with additional anecdotes from others.

There are many books on death and grief and loss. There are blogs where people post stories and websites to other resources and feel part of a greater community in loss. There is even a site to register for dinner parties with others under thirty who have lost loved ones. Many of these additional resources are noted in this book in the Resources section.

The photos of ways to memorialize loved ones are to illustrate what has been done, and may be a springboard for other ideas. While working in suicide prevention, the most-asked question by parents was how to honour their child's memory. This section provides real life responses to that question. A tribute is often seen as a healthy way to grieve, and much thoughtfulness was put into choosing how to honour the loved ones represented in the photos here. They may also give ideas to those working with vulnerable populations, as it makes one consider what a loved one really valued.

One participant from my hospice grief support group suggested that we need a vocabulary for grief. To concur with that sentiment and to ensure clarity, some terms in this book are used as follows:

Loss will be treated as a component of death, with loss and death used synonymously; we know that a sense of loss is experienced with most deaths. These often manifest as feelings experienced in grief. Grief and loss, in all their forms, can be experienced for several other reasons, but the loss associated with a death is generally the most traumatic (Wolfelt, 2016).

A great metaphor for loss is a broken beaded necklace. It breaks and that makes you sad. The beads scatter, and you can't wear it anymore as your necklace. Every once in a while, you find a bead. It makes you remember the necklace, sadly maybe, or with a smile. Either way, the necklace may be gone, but the memory remains.

Grief is the complex mix of feelings that emerge from the loss. It has psychological, physical, cognitive, behavioural, social, cultural, spiritual, and philosophical dimensions.

In short, grief is the deep sorrow or inner turmoil we feel, especially caused by someone's death (Wolfelt, 2016). It could manifest as anger, loneliness, denial, guilt, or a host of emotions combined.

Anticipatory grief, according to Samuel (2018), is loss of a person while the person is still with you. This may be due to a dementia, where one grieves the person that once was although they no longer have the capacity to remember. It could be due to a life-limiting diagnosis or a medical ailment with an unknown prognosis, such as cancer, where the grief begins at the point of diagnosis.

This can be alternatively termed *gradual bereavement* or *prolonged grief.*

Complicated grief is associated with pain that does not subside as time goes by, pain that you feel will only go away if the deceased person could somehow miraculously return.

Complex grief is a past trauma, or repeated loss; a loss without resolution.

Secondary grief is hearing of a loss that brings back the heaviness of one's own loss.

Disenfranchised grief is grief experienced by someone who doesn't feel able to express the loss, due to other circumstances. A person who was having an extramarital relationship with the deceased may feel this.

Mourning is the external display of the feelings of grief (Wolfelt, 2016).

This book is written from a different perspective than others on grief and loss. It is not a guide on what to expect or what to do. It is not one person's triumph over grief. It is a record of ordinary people and their ordinary paths after the extraordinary circumstances of life-altering loss.

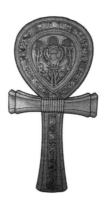

Chapter 1

Cultural and Historical Understanding of Death and Loss Traditions

"What I have learned is that everyone is grieving."

Actor Ricky Gervais, on developing After Life

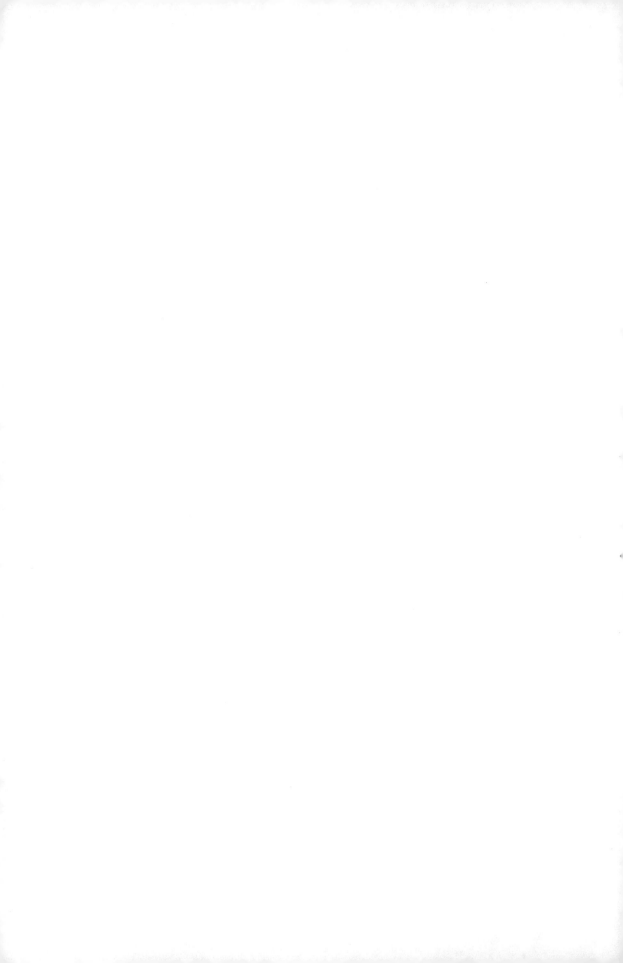

HISTORY AND CULTURE PREAMBLE

Many of the death practices of different countries are steeped deeply in the religious traditions of that country.

In the US and Canada, where we are countries intentionally encompassing myriad cultures, it means there is no one religious tradition upon which to draw. Though in geographic pockets of ethnicity or culture these traditions are still exemplified—New Orleans as an example—generally, the US and Canada ascribe to a generic death tradition. The tradition comes from common wisdom present in modern North American culture about death and dying.

Wearing black historically has been done to let others know of one's bereaved status—that you are in mourning—after the death and for up to two years in various cultures. Wearing mourning dress offered a kind of protection for the bereaved; other people understood at a glance that a person was grieving. Expectations and demands were lowered, a quiet kind of sympathy offered, and even strangers could see that a person was not at their best, due to having suffered a terrible loss (Salisbury, 2019).

Queen Victoria's life was rocked by the death of her beloved husband, Prince Albert. "There is no one to call me Victoria now," she wept, in response to the grinding loss of intimacy, affection, and physical love that she felt (Rappaport, 2012).

Victoria descended into a crippling state of unrelenting grief, and her intense sorrow endured well beyond the usual two years of conventional mourning. She ordered strict observance of mourning clothes for herself and those in her castle, and some of her actions even threatened the monarchy. She mourned Prince Albert for forty years; the only thing of interest to her was her mission to memorialize her husband in perpetuity.

Queen Victoria wore black and slept beside an image of Albert, and she even had a set of clothes laid out for him each morning, right up until her own death in 1901 (Rappaport, 2012).

That tradition of wearing black has been relegated to the funeral now, and is not always practiced even there. Some cultures wear a black armband for one year after the death of a family member, and even several Western sports teams have adopted this practice.

This culture uses euphemisms to replace the term *dying* or *dead* or *died*. *Passed away, lost, went home, is gone* all might be said instead of referring directly to death. Why do we shy away from addressing it head-on? It might be the same reason that we speak in hushed tones about the loved one, or not mention them after the funeral. There is a vulnerability to discussing death. We fear upsetting the people who have lost their loved one. We might then be awkwardly faced with their tears or lack of composure. Or worse, feel like we caused it, when in fact, it is the death that caused the grief. "We know we can't do anything about the death, so why talk about it?" was another rationale given (K. Anderson, personal communication, February 20, 2020). People who visit don't know what to say to give comfort. They may feel at a loss for words. And the scarcity of people visiting after the funeral was noted by most interviewed and anecdotal commenters, noting that "friends scattered" (C. Rogers, personal communication, June 14, 2019) or "I didn't get invited out with any of our couple friends again" (J. Hunter, personal communication, October 23, 2019).

Slow, somber, heavy music such as baroque style or dirges are what we typically think of for funerals (J. Harder, personal communication, November 22, 2019). These were to reflect the emotions of the family members and their loss. A practice of playing popular music, often partnered with a slide show of photos of the deceased, is becoming more common (K. Armstrong, personal communication, September 28, 2018).

Another interesting phrasing of words is about the funeral itself. In the past, no matter how or where it was held, the events were referred to as a *viewing, funeral,* or *wake.* Now, because that conjures up visions of women in black veils sobbing, we say *service,* or *celebration of life.* There may be a distinction made about the building being a crematorium, a church, or a funeral home, or other appropriate location. The city of New Orleans has taken a different approach, with a funeral parade, a joyful event with singing and dancing and lots of brass instruments playing, between the funeral service and graveyard (R. Hunt, personal communication, November 23, 2019).

The Jewish tradition of covering all mirrors in the home reflects a religious rite, rather than a geographic one, as this is practiced in many parts of the US and Canada, not just in Europe. Jewish people also have traditional scriptural readings and a prayer called the *Kaddish* that is always said for the dead.

I was told by a person of Stó:lō Indigenous heritage that in her family, they take away all the photos of the person who has died. They make that loved one's favourite food and burn it with a set of their favourite clothes (J. Jordan, personal communication, January 15, 2019).

It is so interesting to explore the rituals of other cultures. You will note that many of the places discussed below are islands, except Egypt, Mexico, and New Orleans. The practices of the islanders may have been sustained because of the more insular and contained geography. As the world seems to shrink, through the extensive use of social media, these practices may also diminish.

I had the opportunity to tour Egypt in September 2019 for about ten days, and share some of that learning here:

ANCIENT EGYPTIAN CULTURE

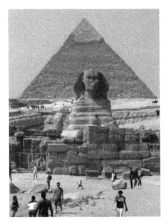

The first written records of death and burial are the Egyptian hieroglyphs. These mentioned the name of the loved one in an enclosed oblong called a *cartouche*, a group of hieroglyph symbols representing the loved one's name and title, and often presented symbolic meaning of the person's life. Fittingly, the greatest architectural monuments of death are the pyramids, where much of this hieroglyph language is displayed (R. Fakhry, personal communication, September 14, 2019).

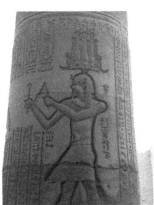

These were mausoleums for the wealthiest people. Although slave labour was used for most other tasks, Egyptians proudly shared that only fellow Egyptians had the engineering ingenuity and ability to build these burial houses. Life on earth was significant as it was the time for people to prepare for the afterlife. This concept was acknowledged at the time of the building of the pyramids, and is still a prevalent belief today, practiced by both Muslim and Christian residents of Egypt. The deeply held religious beliefs were prominent in conversations and spoken of as based in fact rather than faith (R. Fakhry, personal communication, September 14, 2019).

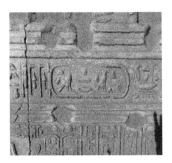

In some cases, live slaves or animals were buried alive in the mausoleums as well, to help direct the deceased into the afterlife. These excesses included mummified bodies, golden sarcophagi and mummified food. Material wealth such as dishes and precious metals and gems were placed in the pyramids as well, as payment for the sins on earth, and to provide for a more glorious afterlife (R. Fakhry, personal communication, September 14, 2019).

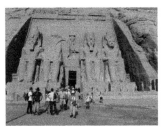

One of the beliefs shared by an Egyptian guide on my tour was the idea that people really die twice. Once their physical bodies can no longer sustain them, they die the first time. Then, when they are no longer remembered and spoken of on earth, they die for the second and final time. It is that belief that made the pharaohs build great edifices, such as the pyramids with prominent cartouches to keep their memory, and by extension, themselves, alive for all time (R. Fakhry, personal communication, September 14, 2019).

MAORI CULTURE

(Due to the COVID-19 pandemic, I did not get to visit New Zealand and speak directly to practitioners, but instead spoke with a former New Zealander in Canada, who travels "home" regularly.)

Maori visit and pray for the person with a life-limiting illness before they die, if possible.

Traditionalists believe that the spirit continues to exist after death and that the deceased will always be a part of the *marae*, or traditional meeting place of the community. Once someone has died, they will go to the spirit world, and a ceremony is done to free the spirit from the body.

The body will not be left alone at any time until it is buried. It will be taken to the traditional meeting place so that all who wish can pay their respects. Family and friends share their grief openly and loudly.

At the funeral, a meal is shared, and singing and storytelling is done about the deceased. The body is usually buried, rather than cremated, to return it to the earth.

The family's house is then blessed to make sure the spirit of the deceased does not remain there. Maori believe the dead should be remembered and respected so the family will regularly visit the grave (J. Kitanga, personal communication, February 24, 2019).

The *Manawa Wera haka* (ceremonial folk chant and dance) is usually performed at funerals or after somebody's death. No weapons are used and the movement is freer than some other haka, in which adherence to precise choreography is expected.

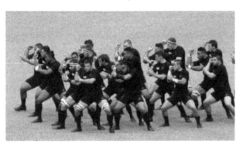

The most famous haka heard internationally is the *Ka Mate* haka. This is the haka performed by the New Zealand rugby team, the All Blacks. The main body of the chant speaks of death and life. The origin of this haka was a celebration of life over death (*Pocket Guide*, n.d.).

TAIWANESE CULTURE

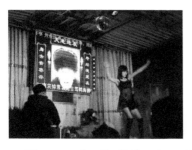

Most people in Taiwan have traditional values based on Confucian ethics. Confucianism stresses duty, loyalty, honour, filial piety, sincerity, and respect for age and seniority. The teachings of Confucius describe the position of the individual in society. Although social class is significant, the teachings stress the obligations of all people toward one another (Taiwan Guide, n.d.).

The prevalent belief systems in Taiwan are a blend of Buddhism, Taoism, and Chinese folk religion, including Chinese ancestral worship, Mazu worship, Wang Ye worship and Zhai Jiao traditions. Still, some traditional values remain strong, including piety toward parents, ancestor worship, a strong emphasis on education and work. The importance of "face" considers a sociological principle that if honour and dignity are lost, there is shame brought onto the individual and family (Taiwan Guide, n.d.).

In may seem incongruous to Canadians, but Taiwanese culture often celebrates funerals with strippers. This is a relatively new phenomenon, started in the 1980s by criminals who ran some of the mortuary businesses. It is thought to invoke a joyful atmosphere to bid farewell to the loved one (Edwards, 2017).

A film has been made about this practice by Marc L Moskowitz, entitled *Dancing for the Dead: Funeral Strippers in Taiwan.*

Dancing at funerals is a ritual that has been evidenced in cultures in South Africa, Ghana, and Madagascar as well (Edwards, 2017).

BALINESE FIRE BURIAL

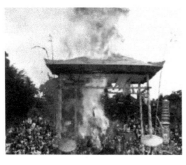

Bali is known as "The Island of the Gods" (https://timetravelbee.com). It is a popular tourist destination. The local people incorporate religious rituals into everyday life. The religious tradition is Bali-Hinduism, a combination of elements of animism, ancestor worship, and Hinduism. People gather at the many temples every evening and for feast days, as well as daily personal rituals, including prayer. Women commonly walk around with trays full of flowers and incense, offering these to the spirits and ancestors. In Balinese Hinduism, nature is considered the source of power, and each element is subject to influence from spirits. Ancestor worship is a very important part of Balinese beliefs and daily activities (https://timetravelbee.com).

The funerary custom combines religion and cremation in a ritual known as the *fire burial*. Influenced by Hindu practices, families send their loved one to re-enter the cycle of reincarnation, enabling the soul to enter the afterlife. There is less sadness associated with the death and no overt mourning, and the people of Bali are more accepting of death and see it as less final (https://timetravelbee.com).

"There are two different sides to everything you see in Bali: the tangible side and the magical one. In Balinese culture, there is no real distinction between the secular and the religious. Therefore, the supernatural is often a part of daily life activities" (https:// timetravelbee.com).

Another place I was privileged to visit and study was New Orleans, Louisiana, in the United States. A web search of "cultures that celebrate death", listed New Orleans first as a city that celebrates death well (https://www.talkdeath.com/cultures-that-celebrate-death/). This was affirmed by tour guide Ron Hunt (R. Hunt, personal communication, November 23, 2019) and indeed is home to the world's death museum! Here is some of the information I gathered there:

NEW ORLEANS CULTURE

There was much talk of death and ghosts throughout the tours of the city of New Orleans. St. Louis Cemetery No. 1 is the oldest in the US, where early French and Italian settlers competed for magnificence in the size of mausoleums contained there (see Chapter 5 for a photo). Amazingly, the remains of over 60,000 people are contained in the structures of this cemetery. Periodically, the remains in the structures are swept into a communal bowl at the bottom of the mausoleum, making room for new bodies to arrive, and be placed in the structure. Name plates of all who are laid to rest in each structure continue to be displayed. It was reiterated by the guides that death was not feared, but instead considered part of life (R. Hunt, personal communication, November 23, 2019).

The voodoo culture is present in many of the discussions of death and dying in New Orleans. It is based on a mash-up of tribal practices brought from Africa by former slaves, and Catholic rituals that were added by the slave owners. Guides emphasized to me that voodoo is not an evil pursuit, as Hollywood portrays it to be (R. Hunt, personal communication, November 23, 2019).

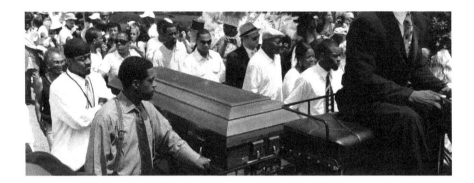

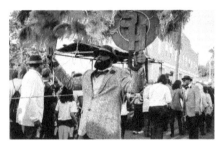

The jazz musical style has given rise to the New Orleans jazz funeral. This style of funeral is a celebration with a huge brass band to commemorate the life of the individual who died. The band meets the family at the church, and the family, mourners, and band all proceed to walk to the cemetery, while singing and clapping and dancing. The procession often starts with the song *When the Saints Go Marching In*. All the people along the route are invited to join in and many do. Traffic stops as the parade walks joyously down the main streets of the city. Residents seem to enjoy the spectacle and clap along.

The ritual of the funeral parade has roots in the African tribal funeral rites of slaves who were forcibly brought to America, and the French military who were tasked with building the city. The parades were meant to help the deceased make the transition from earth to heaven (Edwards, 2017).

"In New Orleans, jazz is a part of everyday life," states blogger Rosy Edwards (2017), "so it stands to reason that it would also be an important part of death."

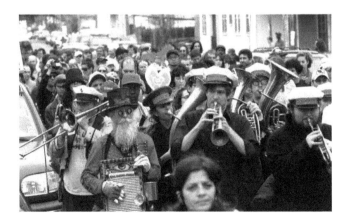

SAMOAN CULTURE

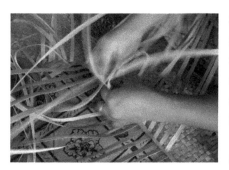

Samoan culture has both ancient and contemporary components to it and these are evident in its funeral traditions and customs. Samoans have a lot of the same roots as other island cultures of the South Pacific, so they have many aspects in common.

The predominant religion in Samoa is Christianity, although ancient myths also coexist with Christianity; this blending of rituals can be seen in funeral customs. They do not abandon their ancient traditions for Christianity, but allow the respective beliefs to be culturally important, especially at the time of death.

Death, in Samoan tradition, is considered "God's will." It has traditionally been believed that Samoans should die at home. Otherwise, it is believed that one's spirit may cause problems for the family. Before the advancement of mortuary science in the South Pacific, the deceased was buried the day after death. Now, it is common to delay funerals for overseas loved ones.

Mats, food, and money are given to the grieving family in a pre-burial ceremony. The importance of mats harkens back to when they served as the currency of the Samoan people. More modern funerals still use the mats for decoration. Appropriate clothing is expected at the funeral, consisting of the lavalava wrap, shirt, tie and jacket with sandals for men, and a muumuu for women.

Burial is practiced, rather than cremation, to return the loved ones to the earth, to allow them to make their journey to the afterlife (https://www.funeralwise.com/customs/samoan/).

MEXICAN TRADITION

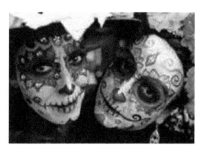

One of the traditions of Mexico and a handful of other Latin countries (for instance, Guatemala) that dates back 3000 years, but has grown in popularity, is the celebrating of Day of the Dead, known locally as *Dia de Los Muertos* (Cordova 2014).

This vivid ritual is commemorated the day after Halloween, when the family visits the cemetery of their loved one. It was originally celebrated in the summer but has moved to November 1 and 2 to merge with All Saints Day and All Souls Day (Cordova, 2014).

The family members clean the grave area, and then throw a party, with flowers, candles, music, tequila, lots of food, and most importantly, a photo of the loved one. They spend time remembering and honouring their dead relative.

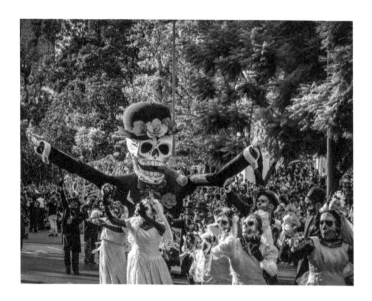

Many see the Day of the Dead as a celebration of life (J. Furtado, personal communication, February 1, 2019). It is thought that this experience helps the people to not be afraid of death. It also ensures the memory of the loved one never ends.

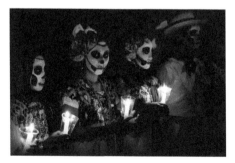

The way it is celebrated has evolved over time, and in different places. It was originally an Aztec Indigenous celebration, and that spiritual practice has merged in southern Mexico with many Christian rituals. This celebration has grown into an artform, gaining an international audience after being featured in recent movies such as *Spectre* and *Coco*, which incorporated the playful aesthetic of sugar masks and dancing skeletons.

"It was a party. Everybody in town would meet at the cemetery to spend time with the dead. I remember seeing all of my friends at the cemetery on that day. It was like a way to honour their life" (J. Furtado, personal communication, February 1, 2019). "You wish this person was here with you. You want to remember this person, and that's why you do it" (O. Balcells, 2014).

Cordoba (2014) stresses that this event does not have fear associated with it, because death is not treated as a sad or scary thing in Mexican tradition. It is normal to not be scared of death but to smile at it.

HISTORY OF HOSPICE CARE

The sick and dying have historically been attended to informally by family and caregivers. This remains the practice in many areas and cultures. The more formalized concept of hospice care dates back to the time of the Crusades. It was recorded by the Roman Catholics of the eleventh century as a way to help the sick and dying, as well as travellers and pilgrims. "The word 'hospice' derives from the Latin word hospes, which means both 'guest' and 'host'" (https://understandhospice.org/brief-history-hospice/).

History tells us that in the mid-nineteenth century Jeanne Garnier set up a facility in Lyon, France that cared for dying people. Prior to this, death had never really been thought about in the health care system—the aim was simply to avoid it (https://understandhospice.org/brief-history-hospice/). Following Jeanne Garnier's legacy, a further six hospices were established in France and New York by 1900. Another hospice was then opened in Dublin, Ireland which helped hospice care spread as far as England.

The modern usage of hospice as a place for, and philosophy of, end-of-life care began with the work of a British physician, nurse, social worker, and writer, Dame Cicely Saunders (Hospice of Holland, 2019). This woman was innovative in the way she thought about caring for the dying, and has influenced much of the philosophy of hospice care today. She added care for the emotional needs of the patient to the care of their physical needs, making the care plan truly humane. She believed in patient-centred care and established the first such centre in London in 1967.

Elizabeth Kubler-Ross's ground-breaking work in 1969, *On Death and Dying*, propelled Saunders's viewpoints. In 1974, the first American hospice was founded in Branford, Connecticut, US, and in 1983, governmental financial support was added (Fisher, 2018). Canadian governments provide partial funding to hospice organizations who adhere to governmental policies, such as euthanasia. Most do extensive fundraising to pay for a variety of programs.

As an example of local services available to the public for free, the Abbotsford Hospice Society (AHS), a partner in the development of this book, provides services that range from grief support in the form of counselling, companions, support groups, and community crisis support, to programs such as The Link, a day program to improve the quality of life for clients (https://www.abbotsfordhospice.org/).

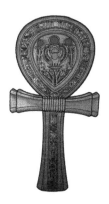

Chapter 2

Stories of Grief and Loss

> **"Tears are the silent language of grief."**
> *Voltaire*

Following are eleven very personal stories of death, grief, and loss. The people interviewed about their experience of losing a loved one graciously shared from their hearts. Some of the stories are longer than others, based on what the speaker was willing to share. Some are more straightforward and some are complex. Some provided advice and some were still looking for answers. Whatever was said, this is one way that those interviewed chose to honour their loved one and have a remembrance of him or her.

After the stories are a few short anecdotes that were enthusiastically given to me to include in this book.

All names and identifying information have been changed in the stories and anecdotes.

ABOUT RUBY, BY BISHOP

Bishop met me at the AHS in October 2019 to share about the loss of his dear wife, Ruby. Bishop seemed a gentle and quiet, mature man. He was polite and deferential in our discussion, and seemed to have a peaceful and contented way about him. When I mentioned this, he said he felt that indeed he was at peace with his life.

Ruby died from cancer, starting in the gallbladder and metastasizing into the liver. She was diagnosed at the end of May. She asked the doctor how long she had and he said four, maybe five months. She spent most of September in hospital and all of October in the hospice, dying Oct 29th. She had been gone from this earth for almost one year when Bishop and I met. Bishop had previously experienced the pain of loss: the deaths of three friends, his parents, and a dear friend, Paul—who was Best Man at his wedding and died of cancer five years later. Ruby's death affected every aspect of his life.

Bishop talked with Ruby to help make plans for her funeral. She picked out the pictures to use, the hymns to sing, and the Bible verses to read. It was a service all about her, the way she wanted it. Bishop was glad to honour Ruby's wishes in this way.

Bishop and Ruby had lived a full and happy life together. He said he didn't think he had any regrets about things done or not done in their lifetimes. They were retired and enjoyed cruising the world over the years. They had many good friends and neighbours. Many of these friends continued to invite Bishop over after Ruby's death, but he sometimes felt like a fifth wheel.

When asked about the routine of his life now, he quoted the Alcoholics Anonymous credo, saying he was living "one day at a time." Bishop was relying on neighbours for support and company, even learning to buy his own clothes by himself. He was learning to cook, as a necessity so he "wouldn't starve." And he was proud to report that he had even learned enough to invite people over for tea. He did feel a loss that he had no one to talk to about the ordinary happenings of the day. He gave the example of when he was watching a veterinary show, and one of the dogs had cancer, and he cried while watching. He wanted to share this with someone.

His face lit up when he talked about the song More, saying, "It was our song!" When I Googled the lyrics, the sweetness of the song fit Bishop so well:

More, by Andy Williams

More than the greatest love the world has known
This is the love I'll give to you alone
More than the simplest words I try to say
I only live to love you more each day

More than you'll never know my arms long to hold you so
My life will be in your keeping, waking, sleeping, laughing, weeping
Longer than always is long, long time
But far beyond forever you'll be mine

I know I never lived before and my heart is very sure
No one else could love you more

When Bishop reviewed his story of the journey, he said he had a new song:

My Heart Will Go On, by Celine Dion

Love can touch us one time
And last for a lifetime
And never let go 'til we're gone

Love was when I loved you
One true time I'd hold to
In my life, we'll always go on

Near, far, wherever you are
I believe that the heart does go on (why does the heart go on?)
Once more, you open the door
And you're here in my heart
And my heart will go on and on

You're here, there's nothing I fear
And I know that my heart will go on
We'll stay forever this way
You are safe in my heart and
My heart will go on and on

When we talked about Ruby's things, he said he didn't part with them quickly. The "stuff sat in boxes in the closet for months."

And although some unhelpful people did tell him to "get over it," he appreciated taking the time to grieve the loss of his beloved. He found great support from the hospice, with one of the nurses even now asking him how he is. He memorialized Ruby by donating to AHS and found they had listed her name on their memorial wall. When I asked what he had gained from this experience of grieving, he jokingly said, "ten pounds." He had lost weight when she was sick, as he spent his time caring for her, but gained it back and more after her death.

He keeps busy now by doing woodwork, and finds taking walks very comforting, sometimes twice a day, to "sort out" his mind. He also sings in a group and has found great support there.

His message for all going through life and loss is: "Don't wait for the future!"

ABOUT CAROLINE, BY DIETRICH

Dietrich came from a great family. He wanted to assure all people reading this that he knows that. But even a great family can have its issues. His issue was about expressing emotions—his family didn't share theirs, so he didn't feel the freedom to express his!

He met Caroline when he was eighteen, and married her at twenty-one. His dad died when Dietrich was twenty, but Dietrich showed no emotion about it, as he thought was expected of him. He became a firefighter, and soon he and Caroline had a child. They had a typical family life, with friends and vacations. His mom died in 2004, after a long, lingering death. Again, he felt and showed no emotion.

Firefighting was a good career, but it didn't allow for emotion, which at the time, he equated with weakness. He said that within the department there was a "herd mentality," meaning that members turned on the weak in the group.

The 9/11 tragedy in New York, and its aftermath, had a dramatic effect on Dietrich, and he decided to retire from the fire department. He went to Fort McMurray to work on the pipeline, but soon found he didn't like being away so much from home.

So, he took a one-year job in Saskatoon where Caroline could come along. Caroline had many stomach issues and other medical concerns. She "died in bed beside me" in 2009, while they were in Saskatchewan. It was an unexpected death, but Dietrich thought he should have seen it coming. He felt he should have seen the signs and have done things to help her. But he hadn't.

He brought her home from Saskatoon and had the service in British Columbia. Then he soon was back at work up north, this time with his brother, Kurt.

In 2012 Dietrich was working on the right-of-way in Dawson Creek. He was lonely, and with a little encouragement from others, decided to try the online dating website Plenty of Fish. It was there he met Nessie, a woman from Quebec.

Nessie was a strong person, that he described as "brash and vivacious." She was a realtor, which he said takes fortitude. Nessie had many unresolved problems though, and was an Alcoholics Anonymous member. He characterized her as "damaged."

She became very sick in 2014. The diagnosis was breast cancer, and it eventually metastasized to her stomach and lungs. After some time, she was feeling better, so they moved in together in Feb 2017, but she was sick again by July. She died 21 March 2018. During that time, Dietrich had focused his whole life on her. "Now what do I do?" he asked. He had given up his life to take care of Nessie.

His brother, Kurt, also died during this time. Dietrich had an Abbotsford Hospice Society companion assigned to him, named Shannon, who helped him deal with the loss, and the lifetime of grief that he had withstood and never processed.

It wasn't until Nessie's death, and his discussions with Shannon, that Dietrich realized he hadn't let himself express the grief he had from all the deaths in his life: his parents, his first wife, and his brother. He had just carried on. He also had the realization that he had Post Traumatic Stress Disorder (PTSD) from all the trauma he had experienced as a firefighter. He learned that talking about it was so helpful. He realized that he had to consider the emotions he had but hadn't acknowledged.

Nessie's two good friends, Rose and Paula, still meet with him for lunch each Wednesday. They worked together with him to clean out Nessie's closet, and those relationships keep her memory alive for him. Nessie's sister, Susan, has become a close friend too. Her support has helped Dietrich greatly.

He has breakfast each Friday with friends from his firefighter days. There have been suicides by many of the 250 guys he worked with in the department. He knows unresolved PTSD has been so harmful to many of them, and though it sounds paradoxical, he knows that Nessie's death helped him to deal with his own PTSD. He stated strongly that "keeping stuff inside, it rots you!"

Dietrich has joined a Meetup Abbotsford group, bought an electric bike, and uses it regularly with a cycling group and on his own. He strongly feels that the physical activity combined with the regular social contact has helped him regain a good life.

ABOUT BART, BY DELANIE

Delanie was interviewed at the University of the Fraser Valley in October. She has a cheerful and self-assured disposition, and is retired from a career in Nursing. She was sharing about her husband of forty-seven years, Bart.

They were snowbirds, travelling extensively in their RV, splitting time between close friends in the US and Mexico, and in Canada. In Abbotsford they lived in a seniors' townhouse complex that had lots of opportunities for social activities and interactions. They kept themselves busy at home and while away.

Bart was diagnosed in November of 2018 with cancer. He became ill with the disease in Feb 2019, and died two months later in April. It was just five months from diagnosis to his death, so not much time, but Delanie looked at it as having "five months for good-byes". They had had a good marriage, and a good relationship, so had no regrets, except of course, it being over too soon.

The main negative emotion that Delanie talked about was the aloneness she felt after Bart's death. She emphatically said no, she didn't think she gained anything from the experience, and she knew she didn't like it! She generally felt supported by her family and friends through Bart's illness and death, though there was some discord with the behaviour of one relative and one friend.

Delanie's children and grandchildren were an immense support to both her and Bart. Mitchell, their oldest son, spent many hours on the phone with Bart during those months. With curious minds, Bart and Mitchell were soulmates in this regard and very much enjoyed discussing ideas, news, politics, science, and human behaviour. Gordon, their youngest, called Delanie one evening in March and told her he was awake in the night and just knew he needed to come and spend some time with his dad. He took the week off from work (with the blessing of his boss) and came over from the island. He left on Friday, and on Saturday Bart went into hospital for the last time.

With their daughter Helena, it was a different connection to Bart, because she had given them grandbabies! Before Bart's diagnosis, and after returning home from Mexico in April, he and Delanie had travelled to Winnipeg for the summer. They came home in September, as Bart had developed a sore shoulder. He was going to follow up with his doctor, but first, Bart insisted on going to Australia to help out Helena and her family. Helena was to start her last six-week practicum for her nursing degree. They could help out, and so off they went. They had an amazing time with their grandsons. Bart bought a folding bike to take. He could go on his bike and meet the boys after school and ride home with them. The boys had two weeks of holiday during this time, and the grand-parents and grandsons went on many adventures. While there, the infamous shoulder continued to be an issue. Once home, the reality that the shoulder problem wasn't going away quickly led to a diagnosis, a week or two after coming home. Once Bart learned he had cancer, Helena came home to Canada immediately and spent a month with her parents before going back to wait for the call.

Delanie felt that the real message of Bart's illness was the strong and unique connection each of the kids had with their dad, and how each, in their own way, found a way to spend significant one-on-one time with Bart to say goodbye.

Bart had a very special bond with his two grandsons in Australia, even though they lived far away. Bart and Delanie went there often. When they were young, Helena came for two and three months at a time to spend time with Delanie and Bart. Each of these young boys, eight and eleven, got up and spoke about their grandfather at his celebration of life. They were not asked, and they did not prepare; they just took a turn. It surprised all of the family as they are so young, but it demonstrated clearly how they loved their Gramps. In turn, Bart had loved those boys as if they were his own.

Since Bart's death, Delanie has chosen to be involved with Abbotsford Hospice Society's weekly Widow's Coffee Drop-In group, as well as join a gym, play pickleball, and take yoga classes. She feels some new independence in her lifestyle, similar to before she was married.

Looking out to the distance, she nostalgically commented that they had a "good relationship, family, and devoted children. We were a team." She felt blessed in the life she had with Bart and all the experiences they had shared. She mused that "it was an easy life, so maybe it was easier to lose him?" They had experienced the togetherness that Murthy (2020) found is so missing in our relationships and culture.

One thing that was extremely meaningful to Delanie was a painting created for her of her family tree, with pictures and names on it: a "tree of life." She treasures that piece of very personal art.

Delanie's final comment was one of gratitude. She felt "fortunate to have had this life with Bart!"

AFTERWORD

The advent of the COVID-19 pandemic has affected Delanie's journey of grieving, giving her time for "lots more reflection." She is still numb, as the process continues, and "as much as I would like this to be over, I know it never will be. This COVID time is difficult in that we cannot move forward in a way we determine. It was much easier when we could immerse ourselves in activities and create a new way of [living]. Still, every day is a new day and we have a choice how to live that day." She feels we have to learn to be our own cheerleader, and find a new purpose.

ABOUT NATASHA, BY GRAHAM

Graham met with me at AHS, to talk about the death of his daughter, Natasha. He presented as a kind, caring man, with deep sadness reflected in his face. He and his first wife had three daughters, Natasha being the youngest. He spoke right away of having not been there to help Natasha, having not connected with her the way he had wished. He felt he had failed as a dad, even as long as six months after her death.

To manage all the emotions that came up for him, he wrote a letter to Natasha, helping him to articulate his feelings. It was a good process for him. When I asked him if this helped his healing, he said he felt he was currently operating at about 60 percent. He said he was outwardly functioning at 100 percent, but really, 40 percent of him was still grieving. His prior experience with grief was recent, when his mom died of cancer fifteen months before, and his dad twenty months before his mom, making three immediate family deaths in almost two years.

Natasha's death was sudden, but not completely unexpected. She was only 34, and had struggled with mental health concerns in the past: Bipolar Disorder, Dissociative Personality Disorder, and addictive behaviours. She had three kids, ages 15, 14, and 4, and was engaged to be married, so it seemed her life was moving in a positive direction. She had had intentional overdoses before, but this one was thought to have been an accident.

Graham learned of Natasha's death from his first wife, Belinda. She called to let him know. He felt disconnected from all the goings on—like he was on the outside looking in.

Graham didn't think he went through the Kubler-Ross stages of grief for Natasha (denial, anger, bargaining, depression, and acceptance), but instead felt those feelings more during his divorce from Belinda. He experienced some strong emotions about Natasha, but couldn't specify which he felt, or when. He may have squashed some feelings at first, but learned this wasn't healthy. He didn't cry right away, but when he did, he was comforted to hear from his first wife, Natasha's mom, that he couldn't have made things better if he had been more actively involved.

He took comfort in family and friends, all huddling around him and letting him lean on them. People allowed him to do and feel as he needed. In particular, two close friends from his church sat with him, quietly. They were compassionate and helped him to recognize his feelings. There were some unhelpful behaviours from others, and some people getting in his space, but he just wrote it off, assuming there were good intentions behind their actions.

Graham was a part of planning for the celebration of life for Natasha. Their family's faith was a real help in that gathering. He was inspired by the saying, "Grief is love with nowhere to go," and shared that with family. He saw a counsellor, and joined the parent's group at AHS. Through those and other actions, he found tools to work out his grief in healthy ways. This was essential for him, and for his career too, since he has started his "dream job" as an administrator at a local church. At first, he felt unqualified to work with others who lost kids, so made it a mission to learn as much as possible, then reach out and help all the families he could.

Two songs that Graham mentioned he found comfort in were I Will Always Love You, written by Dolly Parton and performed by Whitney Houston:

> If I should stay
> Well I would only be in your way
> And so I'll go, and yet I know
> I'll think of you each step of the way
>
> And I will always love you
> I will always love you
>
> Bitter-sweet memories
> That's all I'm taking with me
> Good-bye, please don't cry
> 'Cause we both know that I'm not
> What you need
>
> But I will always love you
> I will always love you
>
> And I hope life, will treat you kind
> And I hope that you have all
> That you ever dreamed of
> Oh I do wish you…

and Mrs. Robinson by Simon & Garfunkel:

> And here's to you, Mrs. Robinson
> Jesus loves you more than you will know
> Whoa, whoa, whoa
> God bless you, please, Mrs. Robinson
> Heaven holds a place for those who pray
> Hey, hey, hey
> Hey, hey, hey
>
> We'd like to know a little bit about you for our files
> We'd like to help you learn to help yourself
> Look around you all you see are sympathetic eyes
> Stroll around the grounds until you feel at home

They both suggest an inevitable sadness.

Natasha's three children are living with their aunt now, Natasha's next oldest sister. She also has four children of her own. Graham shared that Natasha's oldest sister is still often triggered by memories of Natasha.

The lesson that Graham learned was that he had to "cut myself some slack," realizing that he couldn't control the behaviours of another person. Two years later, he finds he is still not functioning at his full capacity and is occasionally blindsided by grief. But he accepts that this is part of the process, and accepts that he's doing the best he can under the circumstances. His second wife, Savanna, has been an incredible source of support and understanding.

A final thought Graham shared was that "grief is a journey" and "you have to do the work."

ABOUT KATHERINE, BY JOCELYN

I met with Jocelyn at UFV to interview her about the loss of her mom. Jocelyn presented as a self-assured middle-aged woman. She is single and raising her three kids. She is momentously proud of her kids and the life she has built for herself and her family. She is employed at Archway Community Services in Abbotsford.

Jocelyn's mom's name was Katherine, and Jocelyn was one of her five children. Katherine was only sixty-seven years old when she died, and Jocelyn pensively mentioned that flowers still make her think of her mom. From our discussion, Jocelyn remembered her mom with great love and honour, which also brought great longing after the loss.

Jocelyn's mom had been at her home on the night before she died, for a birthday party for one of Jocelyn's kids. Two of her kids have close birthdays, so they celebrate them together. Everybody had fun, with games and food and drinks. They all had a good time together with the family.

A couple hours later, her mom called her, saying she had bad heartburn. Jocelyn was tired from work that week, the party, and life in general, so admittedly wasn't as patient as she could have been, but wasn't snarky either. She thought, "I'm already in bed, I just saw you and you were okay, so it couldn't be that bad." Her mom asked her what she could do for the heartburn and Jocelyn suggested apple cider vinegar, trying to give her a natural way to relieve the discomfort. Jocelyn's dad was scared, so she told them to try the apple cider vinegar, and then "she'll be okay." Her parents said that's a good idea and they would try that. There was a suggestion of going to emergency by her dad, but her mom said she's not sitting in the lineup. She just wanted to go to bed.

About half past six the next morning, her dad called, saying "Jocelyn, come over. You need to come." She didn't go immediately, as she had much to do at home to get ready for work at 8:00 a.m. She wasn't concerned, as she had just seen her mom the evening before. She asked what they needed help with, knowing that just a few weeks prior her mom had been sick with kidney and bowel issues, and the doctor had given her medications for these. Her dad added, "Jocelyn don't go to work. Just come." It was weird for her dad to ask this of her, since he knew of her strong work ethic. Nothing entered her mind about it being anything really serious. Her dad, being so concerned for her, didn't want to tell her on the phone that her mom had died, and then have her travel over the bridge from Mission to Abbotsford in that shocked state. So, she continued to get ready for work, but her dad called again. Jocelyn told him she was coming right over, and asked, "What's going on?"

When she arrived at her parents' home, she found it full of people. She saw that her cousins were there. She was angry and confused by the crowd, but continued into the house. She pushed through the people in the hallway and then, there in the dining room, her mom was laying on the ground, just outside of her parents' bedroom. She yelled, "What the fuck is going on?" then noticed the police officer standing right there.

Jocelyn had never been through something like this; her dad and her aunt were there, both crying out. She kept looking around, wondering what was going on here, what was happening. She couldn't understand it. Her mom had passed in the night, so she was already cold and stiff. Jocelyn felt like she was in a Bollywood movie or play, with all the people around, and the wailing sounds. She tried to wake her mom up, yelling her name. It was confusing her—why was her mom on the floor, and what happened? It was the first death of a loved one she had experienced.

Her dad had woken up super early, as usual, and wondered why his wife was not up. He thought maybe she was just tired. He went to wake her, but she wouldn't wake up, so he had family come, and they called 911. The operator said to put her on the hard ground to do CPR, but he wasn't going to try anything.

Jocelyn's mom had never had any heart problems, but doctors said it was a massive heart attack. Jocelyn believes it happened because of the many medications that her mom took daily, and that they messed with her electrolytes. So why was there a police officer there, she wondered. She doesn't know to this day.

Jocelyn regrets not spending more time with her mom. Her daily life of work and children made that difficult at times, but she is grateful for the times they did have together.

She made a lot of calls to everybody out of town, like her kids, having to arrange for some to return from Thailand and Australia. Some of her siblings were more fragile than her, so required extra care, and one had a tumultuous relationship with their mom, which complicated the grieving. One wanted all the siblings to gather together to comfort each other. Jocelyn felt it was unreal how the cousins and families and friends rallied around them. As immediate family, they had to do nothing, really, for the next few days. These extended family members made tea and food for everybody in the house for the next seven days, until the cremation. Jocelyn repeated many times that she will never forget their kindness and care. She didn't know "people could be this wonderful, making food, looking after us. It was amazing—amazing!" She feels like she learned what to do for people in need. She feels it has brought her extended and immediate family closer, and she found it hard to believe that this wonderful positive came from such a negative thing.

In the eastern culture, men don't touch women's feet. But at the funeral home, Jocelyn's dad held her mom's body, and gently touched her feet, repeating, "Please forgive me." It broke Jocelyn's heart to see him hurting.

Preparations for the service were quite intense. Jocelyn's youngest brother took on the responsibility for most of the planning. "He super stepped up to doing the whole funeral arrangements." She added that he was very emotional, "but tried to be strong for the family at the funeral, thankfully."

The service had a beautiful turnout of over 500 people. Jocelyn said she couldn't imagine she would have half as many people at her service as her mom had! It was beautiful but heartbreaking to see how many people loved her mom, that Jocelyn didn't even know. Even the Tim Hortons worker asked about her mom. "I didn't know so much about my mom. There are so many things you don't know about other people! It was really eye-opening!" So many sweet, loving, and really meaningful things were said.

Jocelyn regrets not spending more time with her mom. She recalls often being tired, but yet she made the effort to go see a friend. "But you know, you never know, right? You don't know how much time to share with all the different people in your life." Jocelyn spoke about how moms sacrifice the most and get the least back, saying, "It's kind of a role we get as a mom."

There were things that Jocelyn and her mom didn't get around to doing together. They had talked of a trip to Amsterdam, to the Keukenhof Gardens, where they grow flower bulbs that are shipped all over the world. They did manage to get to the Tulip Festival in Abbotsford, which is a smaller, simpler version of the farm in Amsterdam.

After the service, Jocelyn and her siblings saw her dad as vulnerable. He was not motivated. He lost all zest for living. Through his actions, the kids came to realize that their mom was the strong one of the couple. Their dad wouldn't go for his normal walks. He wouldn't leave his house to go to temple, or for much of anything. For two full months after their mom's passing, Jocelyn and her siblings ensured someone was with their dad each night. She shared that he talked and joked with others, but "I would go over and then we could cry together. It would feel real good—feel so good and just, you know, looking at each other, knowing that we needed a good cry."

Jocelyn found it interesting that her parents actually talked about death. At one point, her mom had said to her dad, "What if I die first?" He replied with, "Don't be dumb. You are way younger than me. Of course, I'm going to die first," because, at the time, he was six years older than she was.

As a family, Jocelyn, her dad, and her five siblings went to India to scatter Katherine's ashes and meet the family there. This was a wonderful experience for Jocelyn, as she felt so much love and care there. It was a truly healing experience for her. She hadn't thought that all the siblings would be able to coordinate their schedules. The trip was an incredible experience for her, having only been there once before. They made arrangements to visit a place at the temple where people scatter ashes. "I felt so ignorant that I don't know the rituals well." But her dad's older brother was so wonderful and loving and caring to them and just treated them like gold. One thing she didn't find helpful in India was that the people around her tried to stop her from crying. They were uncomfortable with it. She learned that you should never discourage a person from crying.

Jocelyn did experience a number of the Kubler-Ross stages of grief. She felt immediate denial, "100 percent," and later, a sadness that led to depression, but even this time was punctuated with laughter. When she acknowledged her struggle, she sought the support of Abbotsford Hospice, and felt gratitude for time she spent with Myra there. Jocelyn did try bargaining, and felt anger, but didn't think she could express it at home, in front of her kids. Instead, she used her car as her safe place.

There has been much learning for Jocelyn from this loss. She feels she appreciates the special people in her life much more than before, and treasures the memories made with them. She takes time to consider these people and keep in touch. Jocelyn shared that she learned we should let our loved ones know that we care about them, and find different ways to show them. She says yes to more things, even when tired. She really thinks she has learned how to care for others in grief. She is taking better care of herself, going to the gym, and eating better, to ensure she will be around for her own kids.

Another thing that wasn't helpful was that her workplace only gave her one week off after her mothers' death. She went back way too early, after a week, feeling a sense of duty. She tried to work, but couldn't focus there. "I was losing my shit I was, like, 'I can't do this!'" Because Jocelyn has a position in which she is responsible for other people's lives, she had to take more time off work, until she could effectively concentrate on her clients again. She wishes employers would allocate more days off following a death, because a week really doesn't make sense.

Jocelyn became bolder, or perhaps took more risks after her mom's death. In one instance, she was walking along the road, and a woman stopped her car and asked for directions to the casino. She was a little lady with a really strong accent. "I told her it was a bit confusing to get to so I just hopped into her car and said I'll take you there." As they drove, Jocelyn was explaining to the woman that her mom had just passed away, and that she didn't have a ride home. She wouldn't normally have said all this, but she was sharing about her loss, and they cried together. "It is a very special memory. It struck me that Mom sent this person to help me. I also heard that a feather falling is supposed to mean that your loved one is looking out for you." Rather than becoming bolder, Jocelyn maybe was just becoming more sensitive.

One of the things she has done is travel. She has visited many places in Europe—Copenhagen, Florence, Venice, Amsterdam—and enjoyed the experiences. She spoke of reading the book *The Year of Yes*, by Shonda Rhimes, and trying to incorporate some of those philosophies into her life.

Jocelyn reflected on her own mortality: "It's great to know that my kids are always going to have those memories of my mom and dad. It's funny though: since Mom passed away, I thought about how I want my kids to remember me!" She hopes that when she passes away, somebody she's done something kind for will speak of the kindness. It will be enough to know that she made a difference in people's lives.

The features of the journey of grief and loss so far, Jocelyn agreed, was that she cares for people more, has grown personally from receiving care, and has grown much closer to her family.

Jocelyn concluded that "It is healing to have love."

ABOUT RICHARD, BY KASSANDRA

Kassandra, interviewed at AHS, was a friendly woman, comfortable in her demeanour.

Kassandra's dad, Richard, had died the prior year, at age sixty-five. He was playing hockey, or more accurately, warming up to play a game. Richard was skating around the ice and suffered a sudden massive heart attack before the game.

He lived in Revelstoke, where the rest of Kassandra's family lives. He was well-liked and personable—perfect traits for someone in the car business, as he was. He could be sarcastic in his humour, but was always helpful to anyone who asked, always there for his family, and had no expectations of others.

Kassandra wasn't there when her dad passed away. All the rest of her family was, so she has some guilt about that. She regrets it, but her relationship with her father was not good at the time of his death. This compounded the guilt she felt. Previously, Kassandra had always been 'Daddy's girl.' Even in her teen years, she was close to him. So, his death while they were alienated was tragic for her. She said, "I had no idea how hard grief is, or how painful."

One thing Kassandra said emphatically was that grieving people suffer in silence. They need time and patience from others. She felt she suffered quietly, saying, "Our society doesn't talk about death or grief, so those who have lost a loved one suffer inside themselves. Reaching out to those grieving means a lot, and just getting to share their story can help so much." For that reason, she was appreciative of the opportunity this interview provided.

When she heard the news, she couldn't believe it was true. Then, soon after, the reality hit her hard. She drove to Revelstoke, all the while on her phone, and was later amazed to recall that she hadn't lost cell service over the Coquihalla Pass—a small blessing! She wished she could reach out to talk to her mom, but their relationship was tense because of the strained relationship Kassandra had with her dad.

Back home in Revelstoke, Kassandra wanted to take control of the many arrangements. She is a natural organizer and planner, so felt she could help that way. There were things, however, that she couldn't accomplish by herself. One thing her father's death has given her is permission to ask for help. She learned that she doesn't have to carry the burden herself, but can reach out to others.

Kassandra felt that she experienced the gamut of emotions through her grief. She described "nonsensical" anxiety, surprising amounts of anger, and sadness, along with guilt. She also mentioned feeling some depression later on, thereby encompassing all of the Kubler-Ross stages of grief. She felt an extensive sense of unfairness that he died so suddenly and so young. They couldn't say goodbye. Eventually though, there was peace for Kassandra.

What has characterized Kassandra's journey so far is that she needed to learn how to cope with her varied and strong emotions in a healthy way. She needed to be okay with not being "over it" when others thought she should be, and she needed to find positive ways to remember her dad. Kassandra said she feels better now, but still not her normal self.

At the time of the interview, the family had not gone through Richard's things. The mere mention of it brought intense anger from some of them. There is the constant thought among the family that "He was such a good person. This is so unfair!"

A nice funeral was held ten days after Richard's death. The vintage car club, of which he was a member, did a car parade through town of all of their antique and restored vehicles. Richard's own collector car was driven by Kassandra, as a "last drive with Dad." She said it is such a beautiful memory, and that she was overwhelmed by such support from the community.

There was a pervasive sense of something unfinished in Kassandra's journey of grief. She felt so badly that she was the only one of the family not there when he died. She missed those final moments with him that all the others had shared, even though he wasn't conscious. So, on the one-year anniversary of his death, Kassandra rented the arena where he died. She invited her family and some friends to join her, took her skates, and skated around the rink. It was a final tribute to Richard, in a place he loved, doing something he loved to do.

Another difficult thing Kassandra had to cope with was the financial burden of taking time off work. Her employer gave her five days of paid leave, but that wasn't enough to manage all the necessary details. She said, unequivocally, that she feels society should offer more time off for grief work.

ABOUT ZANDY, BY LIANE

Liane met with me in her home while her two other children were out and her partner was away on business. Liane was sad. Clearly sad. Burdened. Tired and sad. Her oldest daughter, Zandy, had died nine months prior after a drug overdose. She endured many medical procedures and a long hospital stay after the overdose, before her death in hospital.

Liane was married to Travis at the time, and has two other children, younger than Zandy. They are a physically active family and have a Christian faith base.

We discussed how there are many ways to go through a journey of loss, and so many ways to experience grief. We talked about the fact that it's not a linear thing, as suggested in the Kubler-Ross research, where you work on something, accomplish it, and move on to the next stage. Instead, there is much starting at a stage, and moving to another, then revisiting an earlier one, cycling back again and again.

Due to her career as a high school teacher, Liane understands a lot about young people and that the ones in our society know little about death and dying and grief. They have no life experience with it (we chuckled at that phrasing) and can't handle it when death occurs close to them. People don't understand death, so don't have adequate ways of coping. She said it's like so many things we generally don't talk about in our society, things that make people uncomfortable.

Everybody experiences grief differently. Liane expressed that she felt "every inch of her had tears." She said it was the hardest thing she had ever had to deal with. Everyone was telling her to not cry. Even in her family, she was the most emotional one. People said critical things to her, but she didn't get offended because she was aware that they just didn't understand. They were trying to help.

Zandy, Liane's daughter, didn't have a lot of friends. She had troubles connecting with people, even sometimes with her brother and sister. Liane and Travis didn't know this before, but it became evident after her death. Liane has read a lot of books about death and grief after the fact and realized that Zandy just really felt she didn't fit in, and Liane wonders if there might have been some mental health problems mixed in too, such as anxiety.

Their concerns about Zandy really hit home in November last year. Zandy was "in a state" and that was a clue about her to those around her. She was saying, "I'm taking too many courses," while in her first semester at Simon Fraser University. But Liane felt Zandy needed to apply herself. Zandy wanted to shave it down to fewer classes, less work. School was not going well for her at all, in any of the courses. And yet she had excelled at high school. So, Zandy decided she was not going back to university, forcing Liane and Travis to have a discussion with her about it. Zandy was mad at her parents, and took a bunch of pills in November. A mental health professional consulted with her and gave her a few tactics to help her cope. Her parents couldn't figure out her behaviour because they hadn't insisted she go back to university. They couldn't understand why she was mad at them.

Zandy wasn't happy with her parents, or with being at home at all. She wasn't happy with herself, they realized later. Liane thought they could have a better relationship if they let her live somewhere else, so arrangements were made.

But Zandy didn't see it that way. She may have felt abandoned, or confused, or kicked out, or angry. She was clearly not happy anywhere she was. In retrospect, Liane realizes that Zandy had a drug problem at that time and they did not know. They didn't see her behaviour as desperation, and they didn't know much about drug use. In the state she was in, Zandy decided to overdose by taking over the counter sleeping pills, "a whole pile of acetaminophen and a whole pile of Gravol." Her grandparents were coming to pick her up, since the agreement was she was going to stay with them for a week, just to have a break. They knew that Zandy wasn't getting along with her parents, but they did not know about the drug use. They certainly didn't know she had made a prior suicide attempt.

The grandparents arrived, so Liane woke up Zandy, even though she said she wasn't feeling well. She tended to overdramatize things, so Liane thought it was just her being that way. They sent her on her way with Grandma and Grandpa, throwing up along the way. She even went to school the next day. On Tuesday morning she was still throwing up and said "You better take me to the hospital." Liane remembered getting the call at school from Travis, saying Zandy was in the hospital, and they disagreed on how to proceed. At that point, Liane and Travis didn't know Zandy's illness was because of drugs. Because they were not on good terms with her, they thought that appearing at the hospital might aggravate Zandy. Since Zandy was eighteen, the hospital did not call the parents or tell them what was going on, even though the hospital knew that it was drug use. Liane and Travis did end up going to visit her once, and eventually her drug use became evident. They realized that they needed to get help for Zandy, but also realized that she was an adult and had to want to receive the help.

Liane secured a mental health worker for Zandy through government Ministry of Children and Family Development. They planned to do a six-month course with the worker that included the parents and child. The course was every Tuesday, and the three of them together would do it. It didn't go well, and they went to only two or maybe three of those Tuesday sessions.

On Family Day, February 15, Travis was out of town, and Liane was downstairs with her two younger children. She thought she would go check on Zandy in the bath because she had been in there awhile. Liane found Zandy unconscious and not breathing in the bathtub, so called 911 and gave her CPR. She knew there was a naloxone kit somewhere in the house, but by the time they found it, the paramedics had given her the shot. They walked Zandy to the ambulance, and drove her to the hospital. Again, Liane was not informed explicitly by hospital staff that it was an overdose or that her child had drug issues, although she suspected as much. Being a high school teacher, Liane was aware of the dangers of drugs. Zandy was not admitted to the hospital, which shocked Liane. She was told to take Zandy home and watch her, so she and Travis took turns supervising her, even sleeping in her bed. Liane didn't know how much time she could take off her job to stay home and watch over her daughter.

Looking back, Liane tried to understand Zandy's drug use. From Liane's reading of articles on the internet, she had expected to see withdrawal symptoms, but there were none. She felt like she still didn't have proof of addiction, so thought the drug use was a rare thing. She didn't really know what was going on in Zandy's life, or what to do about it.

Zandy asked and was allowed to go and see her girlfriend for the day. She came back and spoke gently to Liane, saying, "Mom, I just want to thank you so much for letting me go and see her. It just meant so much to me." Zandy said she was going to bed. At some point during the night, she went out for a smoke in front of the house.

Travis and his brother were going to Stanley Park the next day, so his brother and his two boys were there to spend the night. If felt to Liane like everything was just a little off and different.

Early the next morning, Liane's brother-in-law went outside the house and was soon heard yelling, "Call 911!" He had found Zandy outside, unconscious. Travis checked Zandy, but couldn't find a pulse. Liane came downstairs, but couldn't think, and didn't know what to do. "She was just in her bed!" she thought to herself. She also thought "What were you doing out there all night?" She still doesn't know who called 911. Or how long Zandy had been outside in the cold.

Zandy made a gurgling sound, so CPR was started. All the neighbours were there as the ambulance came, and the paramedics worked on her right in the front yard. They took her to Abbotsford Hospital for one night to try to oxygenate her body, but she was then transferred to Vancouver General Hospital. Liane and Travis went home and packed a bag for themselves.

There were operations on Zandy. Each time the doctors suggested one, the family had hope. "They wouldn't recommend to do it if it couldn't work, would they?" Liane and Travis asked themselves. There were so many operations. There was brain function detected, which kept them all hopeful. Due to the night outside in the cold, Zandy's legs had had a lack of circulation, and the damage there was severe. Amputations were done to both limbs. But it was not enough. There was a time when the nurses said that Zandy was reacting to light. But nothing changed.

The doctors spoke to them about every procedure, and they had painful discussions about quality of life for Zandy if she did recover. Her circulation wasn't improving, so more of her legs were cut off. After ten days, they did a full check of her, and eventually, heartbreakingly, declared Zandy dead. Although those were hellish days, Liane said she would go back to them, as there was still hope. She wished she could rewind ten days, when they were all tucked into bed at home.

Liane knew in her head, but it took a long time to reach her heart that her daughter was dead. The shock lasted for a long, long time. The permanence of the situation made it seem so hopeless. Liane said she can't believe these horrible deaths happen to people.

Some people wondered why Zandy had to suffer like that, and go through all the operations. Liane softly said that Zandy needed that time to work things out with Jesus.

Another remark that well-meaning people have made to Liane is that she wouldn't be given more than she can endure. This is a scripture from her faith. She doesn't think she is enduring very well at all. She has gained a lot of weight since Zandy's death. She has also started smoking again. And drinking.

Travis, however, has gone in the opposite direction and is exercising and working out constantly to deal with his pain. He is internalizing about most things in his life. Liane feels she is outwardly struggling more than he is, but he hasn't shared his pain with her.

Liane thinks Travis is also frustrated with her and the way she is grieving. She thinks he is doing all the right things, but here she sits, still feeling so many feelings, and needing to talk about everything over and over again. He doesn't seem to want to talk about it because he's at a different place in his grief journey.

Liane has some regrets around Zandy's celebration of life service. She wasn't in a good place to add what she wanted to what was planned by others. She chided herself for being such a rule follower and just doing what was laid out for her. There were so many fun stories about Zandy that she would have liked to have told, to share Zandy's heart. Or maybe she would have liked to speak directly to Zandy, "up there." Liane knows it was a rushed day and they couldn't do everything. Due to Zandy's love of math and math facts, Liane thought it was cool that the funeral ended up being held on Pi Day, the 14th of March (3.14 is the calculation of what pi is equal to) .

Another difference from Travis, is that Liane has many pictures of Zandy in her phone. It's hard for Liane that the rest of her family doesn't seem to want the memorial things around, but she likes them. It was recommended that she attend the parent support group at AHS, and though she hasn't gained a lot from it, she participates to know she's not alone in this journey. Part of her would like to create a memorial garden in the back of the house, but she hasn't yet, in case she has to move. She may want to get a tattoo, but can't decide what. She knows she will memorialize Zandy at their home in some way. "I have a hard time doing stuff still. I have trouble still making decisions. They tell you not to make so many decisions right away, but I need to do a few things, like for this project, and for some of the research I have to do, I have to go to some places deep inside me." She wants a memorial that is meaningful, but doesn't know what or how to accomplish that. She described experiencing so many feelings, often contradictory, but said she can't keep all the thoughts from going through her mind.

We discussed whether she went through the Kubler-Ross five stages of grief: denial, anger, depression, bargaining, and acceptance. Liane said she absolutely felt denial, like she was living someone else's story, but qualified it and said, "Not outright denial, just shock." She didn't have much anger, but classified it as more irritability with different things. "I'm not even angry at Zandy, you know, even though she did this," she said, but later noticed there was some anger at her. "I just find more of the heavy sadness," she said. Liane is not angry at God either. There was some perplexity about Zandy's sexuality, as she had kissed boys before, but had come out as a lesbian later in her life. She felt her parents may not have responded well to that, with Zandy being their oldest child, and that being their first experience of a child in a relationship. "We didn't really know how to parent, and I know the first child is always treated the strictest, even though she had been around the longest, so deepest in my heart."

Liane didn't think she did any bargaining. She is a pragmatic person, so felt reality was always there. She doesn't think she's at acceptance yet, but knows she has to accept Zandy's death because there is no alternative. She expressed conflicting thoughts again: "I had to accept it because it's our physical reality, but my heart will never let go. I don't want to."

With the realization that the two younger siblings are going to have different memories of Zandy than Liane and Travis, she commented, "Yeah, I'm just glad they've got each other and they're really close." She is concerned, from reading some of the current literature, that the two kids will start experimenting with drugs too. Then she thought out loud and wondered if they already are. She decided, "I don't think so. I really hope not. What more of a lesson can you get?"

A song that was helpful to Liane, especially in the hospital, was Beautifully Broken by Plumb. "Zandy was broken, like the words in that song. It was like it was for her. Broken in her heart because she was using. But then in the hospital her body was broken again. It meant so much."

Zandy's sexuality—identifying as a lesbian—was an issue for her, and thought to have been a trigger for her. She didn't understand it or have peace with it. She also may not have thought her parents accepted it, although they never said that, instead reiterating their love for her. But her mom thought it was a major battle for Zandy. She was "acting angry at God and questioning why she was that way."

As her parents, Liane and Travis knew, even before Zandy shared her sexual identity with them. They worried for her, not knowing much about that world or lifestyle. They were confident, however, that Zandy was a good person, which was all that mattered to them.

When asked about anything she gained from this experience, Liane strongly said, "Weight! I have definitely gained weight!" I mentioned that the average person gains or loses twenty-six pounds in the three months after the death of a close loved one. Other than that, Liane mentioned perspective. She explained how she sees others who have suffered, and are suffering, differently now. She heard about classmates of her kids who had cancer, and she remembered sobbing for three nights straight about it, and couldn't imagine what the families were going through. "I think true empathy is hard," she said. One thing Liane felt was remarkable was how many people are dealing with heaviness and loss. She said we don't realize it, and we might be shopping or getting gas beside someone who is suffering. It is something we don't talk about in this culture. That's why she wants to leave pictures around the house, even though she is aware that some cultures take down all the pictures of the person that's died. There are also cultures that cover up pictures with a black cloth. Even the old traditions of wearing a black armband would let others know. In the Old Testament, they tore their clothes and wore sackcloth and smudged their heads with ashes, like some religions do today for Ash Wednesday. She thought an outward symbol of mourning would be good to have.

"I really don't feel like people feel free to talk about their loved ones or free to talk about the journey after a death," Liane observed. She felt that as people don't talk about their grief, no one really can empathize. "Most people just want to go on with their lives and not talk about such sad things. Yet everyone is going to go through this—losing someone close to them." Her friends wanted to do things for her, but she wished for someone to just sit with the pain with her and her family.

Liane's psychologist recommended Eye Movement Desensitization and Reprocessing, and Liane found it very helpful. This technique was especially useful because she felt a lot of guilt. "The 'what ifs' were just eating at me."

ABOUT BEN, BY MELISSA

Melissa is an articulate woman who lives in Abbotsford, BC. She shared about the loss of her second husband, Ben. They had been married for ten years, splitting most of that time between northern BC and Palm Springs, California. She has experienced many losses that are layered one on top of the other, including the loss of her first husband, and felt that though these events were difficult to go through and live with, they were therapeutic.

We met at her home as her pet was ill and she wanted to be close to him.

In 2018, Ben was diagnosed "out of the blue" with cancer. At the time he was happy, healthy, and fit, adding to the shock. This precipitated their move to Abbotsford from northern BC to be near the cancer centre and Melissa's daughters who live in Mission. A fire in their business added to the trauma of this time in their lives. Making this move meant Melissa was leaving the supportive community of her small town in 100 Mile House, and the community of friends she had developed in Palm Springs. She hasn't yet found her people in Abbotsford, which compounds the loneliness and feelings of loss she is experiencing still. At times she has thought "What's this all for?", "What's next?", and "What am I supposed to do now?" She has experience in community theatre and hopes to get involved in one of Abbotsford's several theatrical groups in the near future.

Common wisdom suggested to Melissa that she not make big decisions soon after Ben's death, but yet she was asked to do so much decision making! She felt she wasn't ready to decide on high-stakes plans, or even day-to-day issues, but she needed to, to follow the typical Western pattern of death, mourning, funeral, move on. She felt some anguish when Ben's son did not come to see him. Melissa's mind was still foggy, and memories of her first husband's passing kept playing in her mind and on emotions too. She made lists and lived off the lists to ensure everything that needed to be done was done. Her own health suffered as a result of her devotion to her ill husband. She attended all the doctor, chemotherapy, and radiation appointments to help remember everything for Ben and to clarify procedures, and feel informed. She emphatically commented that what distressed her is that nobody speaks about the psychological toll of this illness and how to help people navigate the emotions. She felt it would be helpful to have a support person attend those early appointments, to be there for the family. This type of companion is mentioned by Atul Gawande (2014) in his book *Being Mortal*.

A compounding factor for Melissa was the death of her first husband, Lloyd, from cancer, after a long marriage. From that experience, Melissa knew the finality of the diagnosis with Ben. She understood she would be focusing on Ben—his appointments, medications, hospital stays—all the necessary things to keep him comfortable. Supporting his living took over her life. She didn't relive Lloyd's death, but she felt it weighing on her, knowing what to expect, knowing what was ahead, but hoping it would be different. Friends shared recoveries from cancer to help her be hopeful, but she knew the outcome to expect.

The year after the diagnosis was one of appointments, waiting, and hoping. It seemed that the medical care was about the disease and not about Ben. It was a busy time, adjusting arrangements, making new plans, doing everything to keep Ben comfortable, then nothing. There were no offers of help with the emotional toll of his sickness. She felt like a deer caught in the headlights, with all the reports of the physicians, and the questions asked of her. She didn't ask questions as she didn't know what to ask. There was nothing done during his illness to prepare her for the nothingness of after he was gone. This disappointed her greatly, and Melissa feels this is something that could be improved in our social system, by perhaps having a psychologist attend those oncologist meetings that deliver the news of the finality of a life. She wished we would "Stop pretending we'll get out of this alive!"

We talked about the need to look outside of the Western culture to see ways to support grieving people. Here in our Canadian culture, because we don't talk of death, she posited that it impairs the way we deal with it. "It makes it more fearful. Why not set up a way to make it just as normal as the way we're talking here?" We discussed the Mexican commemoration of the Day of the Dead, where families intentionally and actively remember their loved ones that have passed away. We also discussed the hospice as a source of core services.

A further complexity for Melissa was that one of her best friends, Wink, died three weeks after Ben. It changed the course of her grief. After only three weeks as a widow, she felt she needed to be the support person to another widow, instead of being supported herself. The ultimate dilemma happened when Wink's funeral was scheduled on the same date as the scattering of Ben's ashes in 100 Mile House. Melissa desperately wanted to be at both events. After some negotiation, the dates were adjusted so Melissa could attend both, but this added stress. There was a keen sense that her grief was disregarded or less important. She was angry that honouring the loss of Ben was put aside.

Cleaning out Ben's belongings happened with Melissa's move from 100 Mile House to Abbotsford. Having that reason to do it forced her to attend to that task, although it felt like cutting away something she wasn't quite ready to shed. The rest of the move, however was a gift. Their friends, kids, and grandkids all took care of everything connected with the move, down to the detail of a kind friend changing the switch plates in her new home. And the new home became her sanctuary.

Melissa also has to travel to Palm Springs to clean out her place there. She sold it, as she felt it was a place they enjoyed as a couple, and she didn't want to be there as a single woman. She called all the changes that she has been forced to make "mourning for her life."

Ben's death has caused Melissa to consider her own mortality, and what she wants done for her remains. She has read about people having their loved ones made into diamonds, or set on fire, in some cultures. Melissa has told her children, however, that she wants her ashes to be placed into fireworks and shot into the sky.

Melissa shared that she feels we cheat people out of grieving by not talking about illness or death, or not having the courage to mourn.

ABOUT RUPERT, BY PENELOPE

Penelope has experienced lots of grief and loss in her last years. Her friend Candace endured pancreatic cancer, and died in 1993 after two years of fighting for her life, spending seven months in hospice care. Penelope took her to the emergency room eleven times to get a diagnosis. Penelope spent almost all time she had with her friend, and was the one to convince her to go into palliative care, spending months in hospice care. Candace wanted Penelope there all the time, so Penelope spent many nights and weekends there. She was newly divorced, a single mom of two kids, and working full time, but she kept this commitment to her friend.

Two months later, Penelope was diagnosed with diabetes, and she felt that the stress of supporting her friend contributed to this. She thought crying was a weakness, and her family was uncomfortable with emotion, so she just held her illness inside her, which led to a deep depression.

To add to this burden, her dad died from the long and debilitating disease of MS. Her mom passed away soon after. And most recently, a year and a half ago, she lost her beloved husband, Rupert. He died of a combination of health challenges, and had experienced a physical decline over the prior seven years. He had three heart attacks which left him with only 40 percent heart function, kidney failure, and blood clots.

She remembers crying so much, and feeling so overwhelmed and exhausted, saying she couldn't get a grip. Her head kept repeating to her that she could get over this because she's a strong woman. Her daughter gave her insight by saying, "Mom, I don't believe you've been allowed to cry in your lifetime, so go ahead and cry all you want. It's not a show of weakness, rather an important tool in the healing process." She still felt anger at the circumstances of Rupert's illness, and the complicated health care he received. There hadn't seemed to have been a holistic approach, but more of a piece-meal attention to each symptom. They had consulted naturopaths, and fought his illness with pharmaceuticals, but eventually made the decision to let him die. They had been together twenty-six years.

This time of her life had other major changes as well. Penelope retired. Then, after Rupert died in July, she sold their house in Ladysmith and moved to Abbotsford in August. She was sad that he never got to see their new home. It was doubly heartbreaking when, while still in Ladysmith, he took her hand and acknowledged that he knew he wouldn't see their new home.

At first while Rupert was sick, and then again through his death and funeral, there was lots of support from friends for Penelope. But during his long illness and after the funeral, she said "people scattered." She was working full time and caring for Rupert. So, six months prior to his death, she crashed emotionally and went into a major depression.

After Rupert's death, Penelope recognized her need for help. She contacted the Abbotsford Hospice and registered and took the companionship sessions. She then became part of a support group that still meets regularly. One of the things that came up during her exploration of grief was addressing the impact of giving up a son for adoption in her teens. She realized she didn't give herself a chance to grieve that loss, as it "just wasn't done back then." She has concluded that support groups are "vitally important to grief—transformative even."

Penelope realized she started grieving Rupert before his death, during the decline of his health. They couldn't do the things they did before, so it changed her life before his passing. She grieved their lifestyle. She felt it was "brutal to see your loved one suffer." Rupert was a charismatic man who attracted friends. His funeral reflected this. There was lots of laughter and stories at his service because that's who he was. She still has a teddy bear that she calls Rupert Bear that she hugs, and it soothes her. But because of the seven years of illness, medications, caregiving, and appointments, it was a relief when Rupert died.

One of the strengths that Penelope has gained through this journey is resilience. She feels she is stronger emotionally than ever before. She is in tune with her heart and soul which guides her. She has become a very good listener. So often, there was nothing else she could do for Rupert but listen to him. She has learned to ask for help—seeing counsellors, psychologists, and a companion from the hospice. She felt the end of her first marriage started that process of reaching out, but she has worked hard to practice the tools suggested to her by these caring professionals. She feels she is very kind now, realizing that everyone is going through something. Penelope knows that the life experience she now has, though painful, is valuable. She shares it as it is needed to support others. Penelope has a group of long-time friends that "have carried her." She feels that they are "there for her" and closer to her than many of her family members. Still being able to talk about it is good. Her friend from Edmonton came to visit and stayed for a few weeks, which was invaluable support for Penelope.

Penelope spoke of deer staring in through the windows of her home. She heard from friends that nature can sometimes carry our loved ones' souls back to earth, so after a number of these deer sightings, she felt it was Rupert in the deer. She found many reports of this occurrence on the internet, as well as feathers and dimes being reminders that our dearly departed loved ones are looking out for us.

Some of the difficult things she has had to deal with are family issues. Rupert's children hindered her in some of the arrangements, both for the funeral and in the distribution of some of his things. His first wife harassed Penelope before Rupert's death, which added to the stress they experienced daily.

Some of the words said to her that hurt her included: "You're gonna be fine," and "You'll meet someone." She knew she would be fine, eventually. But then when her friend died a month later, Penelope was triggered again in her grief.

What has helped? Being with her twelve-, nine-, and five-year-old grandkids "has been healing!" She realizes now that it's okay to say "I'm feeling good" or "I'm happy."

Her advice to those working with the grieving is:

- Don't judge.
- Let life move forward, and embrace it.
- Laugh and enjoy!
- If you need help, get it.
- Talk about it!

ABOUT JORDAN, BY ROSALIND

Rosalind met for her interview at AHS. She was initially quiet and slow to share, but once we built rapport, she was very open to talking about a very difficult journey she has taken.

Rosalind was sharing about the death of her fiancé, Jordan, who was only forty-nine years old. She and Jordan had been living together for eight years. She painted the picture of him as a fun-loving guy, willing to try anything. He was the life of the party, and always had loads of friends around him, laughing, and having a good time.

On Jan 26th they were riding quads together with a few other friends at Stave Lake. They had stopped for a quick break and something to drink. She was anxious for them to get moving again, so hurried them back onto the quads and the trail. Jordan took off on his as the leader, and at the next turn, inexplicably went head-on into a tree.

There was no cell service there on the trail so it took over thirty minutes for the first responders to arrive to "save him," which is what Rosalind expected. She kept telling him to "wake up" while they waited, but he never regained consciousness. He suffered massive head injuries from the impact and died there on the trail.

The service was held shortly after, and the strongest memory she had from it was the playing of the song *Fare Thee Well*, by The Rankin Family. The loneliness and longing of the song was evident in her face as she talked about the service. The idea of living "in paupers' glory", as is mentioned in the song, has been an unfortunate reality for Rosalind. She may not be a pauper, but she has definitely had financial struggles since Jordan's death. They had bought some property in the Maritimes together and had a plan to move there in the next few years. To pay that mortgage, they had moved into a rental home in Abbotsford, and sunk all their available cash into their East Coast retirement dream. However, without Jordan's monthly income, Rosalind wasn't able to make the monthly mortgage payments. His family stepped in to help with that for a few months, and soon after, due to their financial investment, claimed the property as theirs!

That wasn't the only thing of Jordan's that his family wanted, but it certainly was the most meaningful to Rosalind, and the most valuable. If Jordan's loss was the end of one dream, then the loss of the property was the end of a second dream of hers. His family wanted everything of Jordan's, but gave away his treasured watches and hats. At one point, one of his siblings threatened Rosalind to not interfere. His family took Jordan's ashes and didn't return them to her. Instead, they all went to the property in Nova Scotia and buried the ashes there without telling her. Or inviting her. Since then, the family have stopped all contact with her. This compounded the grieving—losing Jordan, and then this big, strong family.

Rosalind did have some people who supported her well. She said the best thing was when these friends just listened to her. She needed to vent and process the whole tragedy.

She also wished there was someone to help her out financially, as living expenses are challenging on her salary alone.

Living alone has not been a desirable outcome for Rosalind. She has purged the house of Jordan's stuff. She has spent time playing video games to keep herself from thinking of him, and his family's treatment of her. But, she has found herself to be capable in new ways. She was able to hook up their trailer by herself, and sell some of their other recreational vehicles. She killed spiders herself, and was able to jump-start the truck, so felt like she was becoming more and more independent.

Rosalind definitely had regrets about the crash. She was mad at Jordan for being reckless. She was mad at herself for not feeding him while he had a beer during their break. She was mad for pushing him to go so quickly after the break.

Rosalind has created a hand-carved cross to put on the tree that he crashed into, that ended Jordan's life. It is mounted there. When she took her husky to the trail, he reacted as they approached the seventeen kilometre sign near the crash site, as if he knew he suffered a loss there too. When she went to the same trail, sometime later, she found another cross, larger, and mounted higher on the tree, placed there by his family.

From this experience Rosalind feels she has gained courage and strength. It has brought old friendships back into her life, for which she is grateful.

She still feels Jordan's presence around her. She sensed him in the wind storm last January.

ABOUT REBECCA, BY SAMUEL

Samuel spoke to me at AHS about the death of his wife Rebecca. He seemed shaken still by her passing. He spoke very proudly about her, and of the engaging life they had shared. They enjoyed many good times, working and socializing with friends. Prior to their relationship, she had enjoyed a glamorous international career as a model, and received much glory for it.

Rebecca was diagnosed with liver disease, and she died of liver failure eleven months after that diagnosis.

Samuel felt there was false hope given to him and Rebecca at the hospital. He has questions about what was done, if all was done that could have been, and how the medical people decided what procedures to do. The couple had hoped that she could pursue treatment and would get better. At the time of the diagnosis, they changed their lifestyle, quitting all alcohol. They had great hope that this adjustment could reverse the damage to Rebecca's liver and she could recover. But she didn't. They both started attending church, and praying for complete healing for Rebecca. Unfortunately, healing didn't happen.

The cremation was difficult to endure; "raw" was how he felt. It seemed to Samuel that the funeral was putting on a show rather than helping the family mourn.

After Rebecca's death, he was forced to accept the finality of life and death. This prompted him to reflect on the frivolity of life and the seriousness of the afterlife. He is finding himself again. The support they received through church and faith really helped them through her illness and death. Samuel sought help. One step was a class at AHS about coping with grief. Another step for him was the decision to make his bed every day. It was a good step for him that allowed him a small victory each day. He leaves her favourite jacket out in the room, on the made bed, as it reminds him of her.

Samuel feels he is in "loserville," seeing all the families and couples around him, and knowing he is alone. He did make a "sacred promise" to Rebecca to maintain his sobriety, no matter what, and has kept that promise. He wants to do things now that will mean something—things that will help people, perhaps getting involved with the Canadian Liver Foundation.

He has regrets. He wishes they had got sober sooner. He wishes they had had a baby together. He wishes she was still here.

....

As I continued on with my life while writing this book, I had many encounters with people interested in relaying key events of death or loss that they had experienced. Some of these were while I was travelling, while others were at social encounters or over a dinner at a restaurant near home.

ANECDOTES

Ethan is a photographer from Tennessee. I met him and his wife on a guided cruise on the Nile River. He shared about his grandmother, who had always wanted to go to Egypt. To support that dream, Ethan had given her a pair of ankh earrings. Ankh is an Egyptian hieroglyph for *life*; the Egyptians believed that one's earthly journey was only part of an eternal life. As she has now died, he brought the earrings on the trip to Egypt and buried them at some significant ruins so, in a small way, he could fulfill his grandmother's dream.

~

When I spoke about writing this book, Don, of a community Meetup group, said he had a different kind of story to tell. His wife had a debilitating illness that caused her constant pain. She and Don talked, and decided to explore the option of assisted suicide. After much thoughtful conversation with doctors and loved ones, they decided they would proceed with the suicide. Don confided that it was a very difficult time from the point of decision to the actual death. For his wife, there was a sense of peace that she would be out of pain soon. Once she had died, he felt a burden had lifted, but was overcome by huge amounts of guilt. He experiences shaming from some people he tells. He continues to feel angry by this response from people who haven't experienced it and don't understand.

~

Carissa's Aunt Mary was in her 80s, and lived in an assisted living facility, having suffered a stroke. She made a physical recovery, but due to a lack of oxygen, she sustained some brain damage. It changed her personality to one that was gentler and more childlike than before the incident. When the pastor of her church came to visit her one day, he wanted to end with a prayer. He started quoting the 23rd Psalm, and she said it along with him. The line, "Though I walk through the valley of death," was the last she spoke.

~

Rachel and her husband, children, and parents were on vacation in northern BC. They went for a bike ride, but her husband couldn't keep up the pace. She teased him, and eventually they made it back to the cabin, where he collapsed. They called 911 immediately, but being so far from a city or hospital, it took almost an hour for the paramedics to arrive. CPR was done the whole time, with the children gathered around their father's body. He was declared dead soon after. Later, that scene haunted Rachel.

~

Anastasia's husband was a long-haul truck driver. During a trip, he pulled his truck to the side of the road. He suffered a heart attack and was dead before the paramedics arrived. Somehow, he had the wherewithal to pull over his truck while having a fatal heart attack. That thoughtful act may have saved the lives of others on the highway that day.

~

Miley had been heavyset all of her life. She felt it was due to her heritage as both her parents were heavy, as well as being immigrants from a tropical country. When her dad was in his 50s, he started having severe health problems that seemed to have no cure. He died of a combination of these complex illnesses. In her grief, Miley was inspired to set herself on a path to greater health.

~

I met street performers in New Orleans. At the end of the show, they spoke of unity of the races and offered that life is to be lived fully because death can come unexpectedly. They told of losing a close friend and biking buddy to a truck. An art installation (pictured in the memorial photos) is at the intersection where the accident happened, to remind drivers to be aware of bicyclists. Proceeds from their shows went to build the sculpture.

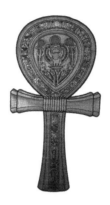

Chapter 3

My Story

> **"The final stage of healing is using what happens to you to help other people."**
> *Gloria Steinem*

THIS OBITUARY FOR MIKE WAS
PUBLISHED IN THE LOCAL NEWSPAPER:

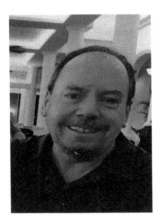

Family was shocked to be informed of Mike's death from a heart attack while he was hiking the highlands of Scotland. He loved to venture into new places, so died doing what he loved. Those missing him at home are his beloved life partner of 41 years, Maple Melder; oldest son Josh, his wife Marnie, and their children Malakhi and Sophia; daughter Amanda and her son Noah; and younger son Calvin.

Mike was a Civil / Structural Engineer since 1985, studying at UC Berkeley and working in California for 10 years. When he returned to Canada he worked for various local and international companies, most recently as a Specialist Engineer for BC Hydro.

Mike was an adventurer, hiking, rock climbing, and mountain climbing while trekking through many different countries of the world, loving his majestic Rockies the most. He was proud to share this love of the outdoors with others, taking his oldest son and oldest grandson on a 7-day trek of the West Coast Trail. He loved gadgets, gear, and technology, and was an inventor, having just recently patented one of his inventions. He was a person of faith, valuing the complexity and simplicity of creation.

It was always an adventure to go places with Mike. He took the high road to Loch Lomond and is now discovering the bonnie banks of heaven.

MY STORY
....

I lost my dear partner of forty-one years in 2018. His name was Michael Joseph Crozier. We met when I was twelve, and he was fourteen, through my next-door neighbour and friend. She, coincidentally, was also Mike's cousin. We began dating two years later, though not exclusively at first. It was quickly apparent to our friends, family, and us that we were deeply in love. Within weeks, Mike showed me how much he loved romance and creative writing by declaring his love in an original poem. That bond we shared built a love story for the ages. Wolfelt (2016) says, "Deep love seems to make life deeply meaningful for soulmates. After a death, the stronger the love that bound two people, the stronger the grief in the survivor."

Mike was an outdoorsy guy. He especially loved the mountains. He climbed mountains, he hiked hills, he hang-glided off of cliffs, he scaled granite faces, he canoed rivers and lakes, he spelunked all the kinds of caves, he camped, he paddle-boarded, and generally explored all that the great outdoors held. He lived an adventurous life, and he died on one of his adventures.

Mike had a long-range plan to walk the El Camino de Santiago from France through Spain in 2020. This hike, however, is a thirty-day pilgrimage and he felt it was an adventure he needed to work up to. The wear and tear on feet, toes, psyche, and joints would be brutal, so he felt that a gradual building up of strength would be best. The plan was to do a one week walk in 2018, two weeks in 2019, and so on. I suggested Mike consider an assisted hike, rather than striking out completely on his own. He had never been to Scotland and thought that would be a great place to explore. To appease me, he found various adventure companies that had packages and chose the cheapest one, though he didn't think he needed the support.

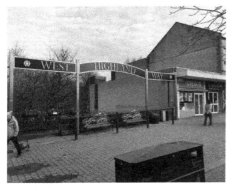

He settled on a ten-day supported walk along the West Highland Way in Scotland, also known as The Way, planned for April 2018. I was all for it. He loved the preparation of gearing up as much as the hike itself, I thought. His Amazon orders kept our postal workers busy.

While on The Way, he texted multiple times daily. We chatted about everything, even while he was half a world away. He complained about his sore feet and not getting a lower bunk in the inn. Some days were many kilometres long, and he had to prepare himself for the grueling toll on his body. He chose to only take pictures on a camera and not send any, so he could enjoy "being in the moment" while he was there. Some of the only ones he sent were of his shoes when he was concerned that he had injured his foot. He thought his one foot had swollen badly, but after he had taken off his hiking boots that evening, he realized that he had accidently put two insoles into his left shoe. He usually had some sort of mishap while on a hike and thought we would get a laugh at his expense yet again. Very mindful of him.

HOW WE FOUND OUT

Six days into Mike's ten-day trip in Scotland, I was home in Canada taking my West Highland Terrier, Wallace (after William Wallace of the movie *Braveheart*), for a walk around my neighbourhood. His breed and Scottish heritage probably influenced Mike's choice of trails, as he was very attached to that eighteen pounds of fur.

While on my walk, I saw a couple of police cars drive onto our street, which is rare. Being curious, I took a shortcut and doubled back toward our cul-de-sac. When I realized they were parking in front of my house, I knew. As I watched the two police officers walk down my driveway, I broke into a sprint (adrenalin brings back old school track team habits) toward the house. Years of Sunday school and church summer camp, brought the Bible scripture Proverbs 3:5 immediately into my head: "Trust in the Lord with all your heart, and don't depend on your own understanding." I did trust the Lord, but I knew. I didn't understand, but I knew.

I met the officers at the street end of my long driveway, and they asked, "Do you know the resident of this house?"

I replied, "I am the resident. How can I help you?" Their faces fell, and the female officer asked if they could come inside. "Sure," I said, but I already knew.

I knew. Somehow, I knew. My stomach was tumbling over and over; my heart was pounding; my brain was racing. Everything else was numb. I calmly opened the front door. I knew, but it couldn't be. He couldn't be gone.

Inside, the cops sat down on the couch. I kept standing. They asked me to sit, but I couldn't. I couldn't hear anything else they said. My mind was scrambling in every direction, thinking every possible extreme thing, hoping I was wrong. My conscious mind came back to the room, and I heard the cops again asking me to sit. "I need a glass of water," I said, and went to the kitchen for a drink. I finally returned and sat on the recliner to hear the life-changing news.

"We received news about a man named Michael Crozier today from Scotland. Do you know him?" Of course I know him, I thought. I've known him for over forty years. "We received an email from an officer there that, just after ten o'clock this morning, Michael died while hiking the West Highland Way in the Highlands of Scotland." He continued, as I said nothing. I felt nothing. There were no tears, just shock. It was 10:10 a.m. right now. He said it happened just after 10:00 a.m.; how could that be? So maybe it hasn't happened. Or won't happen. Maybe they are mistaken. Could this just be a mistake? I knew that Scotland was eight hours ahead, so if he died at 10:15 a.m., then he had been dead for eight hours already. He had been gone eight hours and I didn't know. I flirted with the idea that it was all a horrible case of mistaken identity. Not having had a chance to say a final goodbye made it surreal. This lack stayed with me a long time.

"He is . . . was my . . ." I started shaking my head. How could this be? He was just hiking! "What happened?"

As the officer began to read the email he had received from Scotland, my brain began swimming. I caught individual words . . . "collapsed," "CPR," "air ambulance," "other walkers tried to resuscitate," but I couldn't put it all together. I couldn't imagine the scene a world away that would end with police officers looking uncomfortable in my living room.

He continued reading the email, explaining that the officer in Scotland was trying to locate next of kin because Mike had no information on him except his credit card and Nexus card. He had no address, no phone numbers, no emergency contacts with him. They finally located an address, my address, by putting his name into the Interpol database in Great Britain, after trying the Canadian Embassy, the High Commissioner in Scotland, and Global Affairs Canada.

The email went on: "He was attended immediately by other hikers who performed CPR. Other hikers flagged down a car and went to get an AED from a nearby pub, and a doctor arrived by air ambulance helicopter within 10 minutes. All worked to help him, but he could not be revived, and was pronounced dead on the trail, by the physician." He was "dead before he hit the ground," I was told later by the coroner.

A full investigation was undertaken by a police officer from the nearest town, including interviews with multiple witnesses. "No foul play was found, and it was determined to be an accidental death."

The officers let that sink in for a few minutes, and I started mumbling a bunch of words—they were words that created coherent questions in my head, but were not understandable to the officers. He said that Victims Services had been called for me, and that he and the female officer would be staying with me until they arrived. He then asked if I had any family he could call, or children at home. They asked if there was someone they could call to come and be with me right away, suggesting clergy. I had been raised by devout parents and attended church for much of my life. I have a strong faith. Wolfelt (2016) says that "religion plays an important part in people's attitudes toward death. Whatever the religion, it may act as a buffer against the fear of death. Many religions have a strong focus on the afterlife." I thought I was equipped.

The officers asked if I had children at home. My younger son and daughter were both sleeping. They said they'd like to tell the children. I woke Cal and Amanda, and they joined us in the living room. Amanda's eyes were darting back and forth from me to the cops. She immediately became emotional, never reacting well when police were around. She was suspicious of police from her teenage years.

The kids sat down, and the male officer said he had something to share with them, and he gently told them of Mike's death. Amanda's immediate response was anguished, loud crying with big tears dripping to the hardwood floor. Cal sat up with perfect posture and was quietly taking it all in.

The officer then relayed the email from Scottish police officer Iona Frickleton to which, at the sound of her name, my son Cal said, "Isn't that quaint." We all laughed and then, in the next moment, felt awkward for laughing, but it had relieved so much tension. Iona was an officer from the Killin Police Detachment (another snicker). That was the first of many laughs and smiles we had through this experience and in remembering Mike. The officer asked if they had questions. I am sure they did, but they didn't say anything. He let us know that Officer Frickleton would like to speak to us by phone, so he gave me a copy of the email with her contact information on it. He offered some small talk to the kids as we all processed the life-changing news of Mike's death.

Iona proved to be a godsend, calling me every night at midnight for two weeks, which was 8:00 a.m. for her, when she was beginning her shift. She kept me informed, and was incredibly sensitive and caring. I felt like I had an ally in her.

I had to call my older son, Josh, to inform him. He was so close to Mike; he would be devastated. I called him at work, and since I never did that, he knew immediately that something was wrong. He knew. Just like I knew. I asked him to sit down, and he said he was. His only comment was "I'll be right there." He lives and works about forty minutes away from me, and the emotion in his voice made me ask if he was okay to drive. He said he was and would be right over. In reality, he told his boss what had happened, and drove immediately to pick up his children at their schools. He told each of them and then headed to his wife's school, where she taught kindergarten. She called him because she had just received a bizarre text from his boss, saying how sorry he was, and that he was worried for Josh. He had to tell his wife over the phone, knowing that she would be alone with the news for at least ten minutes before she would be able to see him. He had not planned for her to find out this way, as he knew this would be devastating amid the 20 five-year-olds in her charge.

MY FIRST REALIZATION OF THE CHANGES AHEAD

Mitch Albom (2002) has famously said, "Death ends a life, not a relationship."

While the police officers were in my living room, waiting for my son and his family to arrive so that my children and grandchildren were all gathered before they left, I sat back in a chair, putting my feet up as I reclined. I saw my toenails and started laughing. "Who is going to paint my toes now?" I wondered out loud. Mike had always enjoyed painting my toes, and I loved him doing it. Both children quickly said, "You can get a pedicure any time", and they did follow through, buying me a pedicure gift certificate for Mother's Day the next month. It was such a trivial thing, to worry about my toenails, but it was the first realization of all the changes ahead. Wolfelt (2016) says partners "imbue even the most mundane routines with a specialness and privilege."

After that, I went to a salon for mani-pedis. It was nice to have that kind of luxury and pampering. But my fingernails were getting weaker due to the shellac and my toes were showing less and less as fall approached. So, five months after, I decided that I would do my own nails again. It was such a small thing, but it meant so much to me—I wasn't depending on Mike, or anyone else, to take care of this small detail. This was a turning point for me, a new path, a signpost on my journey.

The officers left the house and waited outside in their cars for the Victim Services people. I know these folks are well-meaning, but they handed me a manila envelope with papers in it and asked me how I was. Trite. Banal. Cliché. What did they expect me to say? I thought how ineffective a program that was, at least for me. They told me about the hospice and their grief groups—I said that I had done some training for them. I clearly didn't feel I would get any help from them. Little did I know how much I would lean on the supports provided by the hospice later on.

Josh and family exploded through our front door. Josh and Marnie were both calm at first, and then sobbing when they hugged me. I didn't let go of Josh for a long time; I couldn't, and when I did, he didn't let go of me. He is truly his father's son. He loves Mike as much as I do.

I went through what I knew again, told the story again. I hugged my grandkids tight. Probably too tight. I needed them close. I tried to fix them something to eat. Any comfort would help, I thought.

I am strong—physically, mentally, socially, spiritually, and emotionally. I always have been. I am accomplished academically, holding seven credentials. I have a responsible career with high status. I live a life of privilege with a middle-high class income. I have good friends that I have known for over fifty years, as well as some newer found friends. I have wonderful children that care about me as much as I care about them. I feel loved. People often look to me because I can help them. But this time, this circumstance, people were looking at me to need the help, to need a shoulder or a tissue. "I'm fine," I said so many times. Fine! I was at first.

Our society creates socially acceptable responses to situations; "I'm fine" is one of those. It really becomes meaningless. Another response I found meaningless was "I'm sorry." People say it by convention, without really feeling sorry. It is just what we are supposed to say. I heard it so many times, and thanked the person for trying to be considerate. But deep down, I know they didn't feel sorrow. I try to say something more meaningful when confronted with the news of a loss. If I wish to express emotion, I check myself for what I am feeling and articulate that. If I wish to empathize, I say that.

Or more often, I say that I can't imagine all that the other person is experiencing. We all face grief differently so I don't think I can ever truly know their heartache.

I wondered later about prescience, and the possibility that someone knows ahead of time that they are going to die. Mike had said goodbye to me three times before his trip. Prescience is defined as the fact of knowing something in advance; foreknowledge. I now believe in this concept. Before Mike left for Scotland, he said his initial goodbye as he always did, with a hug, kiss, and an "I love you," while looking deep into my eyes. I returned the love. Then he went out to his car. About fifteen minutes later, when I was in the kitchen making breakfast for the kids, he came back in and grabbed my hands in a dance posture, and waltzed me around our kitchen island. We had been taking ballroom dance lessons, but this still was unusual behaviour for him. It made me laugh. I asked what he was doing, and he just restated that he loved me. He kissed me goodbye again, and said "I love you" again, looking at me as he always did when we danced. He then returned to the garage to leave. Another fifteen minutes, and I was in the foyer of the house, holding my newborn grandson and talking to my daughter. Mike waltzed in (not literally) and I said, "You're still here?" He didn't respond but instead grabbed my face with both hands and kissed me deeply, forever. This time, he hugged me so tightly and whispered, "I just want you to know that I will always love you," and left for the last time. It was as if he knew it was the last time we would see each other.

TELLING OTHERS

I realized that I needed to inform people about my tragedy. I tried to make a list of whom I needed to call or message. But I couldn't call anyone. I was supposed to be at work in a couple hours to invigilate the work of some students. I called and left messages for a colleague and for my dean, but the idea of calling friends and family made me feel so fragile. I just couldn't. So, my dear, dear daughter-in-law swung into action. She took my phone and texted and emailed people, calling others. She asked one person of a group to notify the others. For instance, my sister was asked to contact all our relatives. My oldest friend, Carolyn, replied, "I'll be on the next ferry over." She arrived the next day and stayed for a week. She was a voice of reason in all the craziness of planning. I was so fortunate to have a person like that in my life and at my side.

Marnie, my daughter-in-law, looked up funeral places, organized the food that kept arriving, displayed the flowers and watered them, and kept everything running. We all need a Marnie in our life, and especially in a time of loss and upheaval.

We have a group of five families that we visit with twice a year, that I have lovingly called the Tofino Family. That is because we try to go to Tofino once each year together and then to Victoria for New Year's. These people all showed up on a Saturday after

Mike's death. They brought food and love and hugs and wonderful company. We shared many laughs and tears. They all showed up later on for the funeral too, even though so many live far away.

I felt I should call Mike's sister, as they had just lost their dad two months prior (his mom predeceased him by forty-five years), so there was only his sister left in his immediate family. She did not react well. She somehow made his loss about her. She said to me, "I knew he shouldn't go. I had a dream about it." I then started to tell her the details I knew, but she broke in and said, "You're too young to be a widow." I didn't even realize that was my new moniker. I was now *a widow*. I told her I had to go and hung up. More thoughts to process, more new roles to learn.

Fine. I was fine. All that day and in those days to come, people came by. Many dropped off groceries. I was watchful, too, trying not to look teary, knowing that if I was, everyone around me would break down and cry. I hugged people who seemed quiet. I sat with those who looked down. I took the puppy, Wallace, to many to let him lick them and make them smile.

I cried still, but privately. I cried in the shower. I intentionally cried in the shower. It masks the tears; it dilutes the tears. My oldest friend said she cried in the tub—same idea. I decided, however, that if I ever felt like crying, I would. No apologies, no questions asked! So when See You Again by Charlie Puth ("It's been a long day without you, my friend. And I'll tell you all about it when I see you again. We've come a long way from where we began. Oh I'll tell you all about it when I see you again. I know you are in a better place . . .") played on the radio, I pulled the car over and cried by the side of the road. Or when I opened the hall closet and saw all the jackets and coats that he had lovingly bought and used, I cried. When I drove home with Wallace, the dog in the car, and the dog saw Mike's car parked on the road, and started jumping and scratching at the window, trying to get to Mike, I cried. I cried again, feeling Wallace's missing as he sat by the back door at six o'clock in the evening, waiting for Mike to walk in from work. Or when I found a card from four years before, from my birthday trip to Tahiti, where he wrote of looking forward to the rest of our lives to explore beautiful places like that; I cried that we didn't even have five more years. Or, or, or . . .

FIRST MELTDOWN

That first afternoon my grandson noticed that the garbage was full. I walked into the kitchen to deal with it. I just stood there beside the garbage can, immobilized. I didn't know what to do. I didn't know where the garbage bags were, or when garbage day was, or how many garbage bags we were allowed to put out for collection. I felt so helpless. I started crying because of garbage. Yep, garbage made me cry. My older son quickly intervened. He said he'd take care of it and not to worry. Such was my first meltdown, but it wasn't the last. I said thanks and walked away from the garbage can, while wondering what I was going to do the next week on garbage day.

And so began my journey into sudden and all-encompassing loss.

How was I feeling? That was the incessant question. I wasn't feeling anything, really. But people didn't like that answer. I felt numb. I had no feeling. Looking back on those first days and weeks, I felt like a zombie, going through habits rather than acting like a fully rational being. I could converse with people, mostly retelling the sad story.

And how that retelling was a dichotomy. It felt good to talk about Mike, about his outdoor experiences, and know that others were interested to hear about the circumstances. But it was also a blow, every single time, when I realized that the end of the story meant that he was dead. That it was more than a story for me; instead a change in my entire life.

When I finally took time to reflect, I realized I felt off balance—off balance enough to bump into walls, to lean to one side. I was listing to the right. "Chaos replaces peace and calm," according to Wolfelt (2016). When I used the term *unbalanced* to describe how I felt to my friend, she said, "Of course. You have lost your left arm." That was the one I put around him. So, I was missing a piece of me. My left arm, and part of my heart.

"MIRACLE MOMENTS"

HIS PHONE

To prepare for this trip to Scotland, Mike had been hiking regularly near our home. Three days before he left, he came home from a two-hour hike, stripped off his sweaty clothes in the laundry room, threw them directly into the washer, and turned it on. Later, when he was looking for his cell phone, our daughter found it in the washer with his clothes, not functioning. Immediately he put it into a bag of rice (as the internet suggested), but to no avail. It wouldn't turn on. He tried taking it to a phone repair expert, but even that person couldn't do anything for him. So, he went and bought a new phone for his trip, leaving the old one at home.

After he was gone, we realized that we didn't have the passwords to his computer or business accounts. We didn't know his credit card number or his passport number. I knew he had a password keeper app on his old, damaged phone. While looking through his office for any of the personal information that authorities were looking for, my younger son and daughter-in-law found his old phone, still sitting in the bag of rice. They thought they would see if they could coax the old phone to share its secrets, and decided to just plug it in to see if it would respond. Within minutes, the screen came to life! It took a lot of lock outs and guessing to get into the phone itself, and even more trying to guess at passwords to get into the app that had the password information. Once they finally got in, they printed off all the info in the password keeper, and used it to open his computer. The phone worked for two hours—just enough time for them to find a majority of the personal information that was needed, and after that, it never turned on again. We felt like it was a God moment.

HIS CAR

Mike had flown from Seattle to Glasgow, Scotland. His car was still parked in Seattle. The difficulty was that we didn't know where in Seattle. We knew it was in a long-term parking lot, but which one? Our Tofino family friends in Seattle volunteered to go and search all the lots for his car. This seemed like a Herculean task. After being able to get information from Mike's old phone, we were able to use his credit card number to log onto his online banking. From there, we were able to view his credit card statement, that just happened to have a phone number attached to the charge for his parking. We called the number and through it, went to a call centre in New York, and were able to get the name of the lot. We then appealed to our newly friended police officer in Scotland, Iona Frickleton, to see if she could locate any information from Mike's belongings that would help us in our search. She sent pictures of all the paperwork in his backpack, that had been stored in their police station. They were all in evidence bags, which was a little creepy, but that gave us the parking receipt which told us the stall number his car was in. This proved invaluable. We made the trek through Seattle and back, and though we worried about it, we had no problems at the border. This was another God moment for us.

BEING A FOREIGN NATIONAL

One of the interesting and probably little-known things about dying in a country in which you are not a citizen is that you then become a foreign national, and different rules and processes apply. One of these processes was that the Canadian Embassy in England was involved and called our house. The High Commissioner's office of Canada in Scotland also was in touch with us. The most helpful of these governmental organizations was Global Affairs Canada (GAC). I was assigned a representative from their office, and he kept in regular contact with me. When some places wouldn't accept the form from Scotland that officially stated Mike's death, GAC let them know it was to be accepted as they would a Canadian death certificate. They also translated some of the terms used in the UK that are different from those in Canada, such as *procurator fiscal*, rather than *coroner*.

Mike's body was taken from the West Highland Way trail to the closest hospital. Then it was turned over to the procurator fiscal (who so graciously called me to read the report as soon as it was done), and then to a funeral home in a different city. From there, it went to the crematorium in a different town. Finally, he had to be taken to the airport for return to Canada. All of this transporting was generously done by the funeral director, Ross Anderson. He became a regular on the phone every morning at 8:00 a.m., informing me of what was happening there. He showed great patience, empathy, and understanding when faced with all my questions. This process of repatriating Mike to Canada took almost a month to complete.

The one thing that Ross couldn't fully facilitate was the return of all of Mike's belongings. Most of them were flown home, but nothing with a battery could be sent by air, unaccompanied by a person. These items, such as his digital camera, car key fob, cell phone, and watch could only travel with a person. I was unsure what to do. As it turned out, the mother of one of our Tofino family members, Greg, was in Scotland at the time. Greg asked her if she would travel with Mike's electronics and she agreed. Ross then suggested he would drive these things all the way to Glasgow to hand them over to Greg's mom. This happened a month later, but just getting these articles back at all was thought to be another piece of Godly intervention. In one of the cases was a very special Celtic ring that had been custom-made for him in Ireland, and I treasured having that. None of this happened quickly. Dealing with people an ocean away, who do things according to their customs and laws was not easy.

The British Embassy contacted the Canadian Embassy, and they in turn contacted GAC who finally contacted me about another matter. The British Embassy wondered if they could forward an email to me that was written by a couple fellow hikers who were on the West Highland Way trail with Mike.

I said, "Of course," and the three pages I received were a poetically written account of conversations Mike had had with John and John, two Scottish men also hiking on The Way. They had met up off and on with Mike in the four days on the trail in the inns for overnights, in the pubs, and in the bothies. They recounted stories told by Mike about his love for his family, for his life, and especially for me. What a gift that they took the time to write and then took the time to locate how to get the message to me.

I was, and continue to be, overwhelmed by the help and care that was provided to me. There are so many wonderful people in this world!

FINANCIAL ASPECTS

People say not to make any decisions for at least a year after the loss of a partner. Yet every time I turned around, someone was asking for me to decide something. Do you want to have an annuity or a monthly payment from his work pension? How do you want to invest? Are there other insurances? Is your name included on all the assets? All the financial changes required decisions. And I couldn't wait a year to do them. In just one week I had five different investment companies contact me (How did they get my phone number?) to help me invest my money with them.

Mike earned a considerable amount more money than I did per month. He had worked for a private company that paid him well at first, but his salary didn't go up regularly, although their profits did. He did receive bonuses and profit-sharing, but had no pension. When they unceremoniously laid him off, with a ridiculous plan called a *working severance*, I saw it as a blessing in disguise. A power company came looking for him and provided a well-respected career opportunity in a large corporation owned by the government. They paid him better than the private company and gave him seven weeks of holidays each year. (He said he needed that vacation as the work wasn't as creative as he liked.) Plus, they gave him a pension.

When he died, he obviously stopped working and stopped receiving the paycheck. Even though my household debts remained the same, my monthly income plunged to less than half of what it had been. This, again, was not something I had ever thought about before. I suddenly realized I'd have to live on a budget!

With suggestions from my very careful daughter-in-law, I did work out a budget based on my salary alone, and I found that even with careful living, I was about $500.00 short per month. Yes, I was living the lifestyle to which I'd become accustomed with two professional level salaries. That's when the people from Canada Pension Plan survivor's benefit informed me they would be paying me $589 a month for the rest of my life—that's about another twenty-seven years by their estimates, and enough to meet my monthly budget. Mike's career was over thirty years, most of it with a six-figure annual income, and out of all those contributions, I get this calculated, actuarial amount. It was a blessing and it met my monthly needs. Money seemed so trivial and unimportant—so insufficient a return for all I had lost.

Life insurance. Ironic. What a name. Like anyone could insure that we would have a life. It really is death insurance. These were the dark thoughts in my mind. Now I recognize that having life insurance is a great thing. As a couple, we never put much thought into it, because, honestly, we didn't really contemplate death. It's not like we felt we were immortal like teenagers do, but we believed in "living for today" (not for April 18th, 2018) and living fully. That's why we had little savings. That is why we used our healthy line of credit. We lived well and so did our family. When I checked and realized there was life insurance on the mortgage, I was surprised what that meant.

The life insurance from his work, my work, and our private plan came through too. I felt a little greedy, begrudging the fact that there was a form for an additional $250,000.00 in life insurance, signed, and on his desk in our den. He just would have had to mail it in the prior two months since it was dated, but he hadn't. The money couldn't make up for the loss.

When I received the first check from our personal insurance, in person, I was thankful, and a little blown away. It was the biggest cheque I had ever had in my hands, yet my only thought was, "Is this the value of a person? Is that money the value of a life? Is that what Mike's life was worth?" I pondered that too much, so much so that I couldn't bear to cash or deposit the check. It seemed too final. I couldn't get my head around that, or past it. I carried that cheque with me for days, weeks. Finally, during a meeting about a different matter, my personal banker, who was so incredibly helpful, asked me if there was anything else I needed him to do for me. Without words, and with tears rolling down my face, I handed him the cheque. It wasn't easy to relinquish it to him.

FUNERAL, SERVICE, OR CELEBRATION OF LIFE

A large part of having a death in the family is the planning of the funeral, memorial service, celebration of life, or whatever you wish to call it.

I had helped plan my father's and then mother's services, but this was different. I felt it was up to me to share Mike's life and death in a way that would represent him well, and that he would have appreciated. But what was that? Again, we had never thought about our own deaths, or discussed what we wanted said about us in memorial, so I was on my own to choose and plan how to encapsulate the life of another soul. It is not like I had to do it all, as all the family was ready to help. But as an educator, I knew we wanted a central theme to align all aspects of the service.

I will admit it's weird to say, but I loved Mike's funeral, or service, or celebration of life. It shared about him as an adventurer. People who had worked with him for over twenty years said they didn't know all that about him. It clearly shared his love for his family. All the kids participated and even a couple of the grandkids. Dear friends from our life in California came for the service, some speaking or singing. Other local friends participated with their gifts of music or prayer. His favourite songs were a background for the slide show, that I couldn't watch, which played behind as the eulogy was given. We had pictures and memorabilia of his life on tables, and a place for attenders to write their memories. An adaptive paddling society that Mike had donated time to was chosen as the charity to support for those who wished to donate in his name, and they presented a significant plaque as a tribute to his contribution.

I had asked for one hundred chairs to be put out for attenders. The pastor said he would put out 150, but leave more in case. In all, over 250 people attended the service.

And there were flowers. So many flowers. They were beautiful gifts, wonderful remembrances. They brought colourful life to the service and to our home. But they made me sadder. They needed care when I could barely care for everything else. And they, too, died too soon.

UNHELPFUL THINGS

Interestingly, there were places in Canada that would not accept the certificate of death issued in Scotland. Rather, they would only honour the Canadian death certificate that they recognized. GAC stepped in to help, connecting with the agencies to let them know that the Scottish document was legitimate.

I had to try to remotely organize all the affairs for Mike's "funeral" in Scotland, before his cremation. I was fortunate to have the caring support of Ross Anderson, owner of a funeral home there, who was able to manage international funerals. He took care of the arrangements after asking my wishes, and I willingly paid him for his services. However, Canadian rules required that I also pay for the services of a funeral home in Canada, even though I didn't use their services at all. But via a funeral home was the only way to receive Mike's remains that were shipped by Ross in Scotland. I didn't need the extra cost or intermediary company, but was forced by rules.

I felt it necessary to share the news of Mike's death with my closest neighbours. They were supportive, offering help and attending the funeral service. I also told one neighbour who was close by proximity, although only an acquaintance. She felt bad to hear the news, particularly because she had been upset with Mike the last time she spoke to him. While we were away from our home one day, making arrangements, she surrounded a rectangular patch of garden in rocks, with Mike's name written on a large stone placed at the head, with some flowering plants at the back. When I drove into my driveway, I was shocked to see what looked like a grave! Right beside my driveway! I didn't know who did it or why, but it absolutely stopped me in my tracks. My daughter-in-law, following behind me in her own car, jumped into action, saying "This isn't happening," and throwing the stones into a pile to the side, including the named "headstone," making it just a driveway once again.

My workplace was kind enough to buy me a plant in remembrance of Mike. What was interesting to me was that none of them visited or brought it to me. They asked me to pick up the plant myself from my office. Some did email or text. Two colleagues from my department came for the funeral. However, there was a huge amount of support from faculty, administration, and staff from other departments, and many students and grads came. It was uplifting for me to see all those who came to support me and I will always be grateful for them!

Related to my employment, I was met by our director of HR to discuss my loss of Mike. He compassionately told me to take all the time I needed. I shared with him that I had already scheduled a semester off from work so would be back in eight months. That time to process everything gave me great peace. However, for others who work there, the collective agreement we have grants a leave of absence, with pay, for up to a total of seven work days per calendar year for bereavement (UFV, 2016). I couldn't imagine going back to work ten days after Mike died. We hadn't even had the celebration of life yet!

Fourteen months after Mike died, in June 2019, a colleague, who had attended the funeral, asked me to share the details of what happened, as we were planning a work-related trip to Scotland. I started telling her, but realized I couldn't remember several of the details. My forgetting was not helpful to me, as I felt like I had let Mike down—had lost something very personal and precious. I was determined to record all I could recall, in hopes of honouring him, and perhaps to help in comforting others. That was the genesis of this book.

CARING FOR THE PRACTICAL: THE HOUSE

Was the universe telling me to move? Weeks after Mike died, the garage door stopped closing. I forced it, then it would not open again. We soon found that the hot water tank needed replacing or ran the risk of bursting. The air conditioning function of the heat pump was not cooling and we were told it was because the air ducts needed cleaning out. Then the main floor powder room toilet was not flushing while the one in the master suite was plugged and flooded. The dryer needed replacing, and the dishwasher stopped working. All of this was in the three months after. So, ten months after, I moved!

WHAT ABOUT HIS STUFF

Many people, for just as many reasons, don't want to get rid of their loved one's things. That is, when do you clean out their closet? Or give away their toys? When is the right time?

I was fortunate to have my grandkids do this with me. I sat on the futon as one kid went through the closet and the other went through the three dressers of clothes. They packed most to be given to charity, but kept a few things for themselves, or their dad, or for me. I gave away his Apple watch to a business partner of his, and his rings, watches, coats, and knives to any of the family who wanted them.

What I found is that the right time is when you are ready to part with the stuff, and only you will know when that is.

THE MUNDANE

....

When I consider the things that I have learned from this experience, one is an appreciation for the mundane. I used to hope for excitement and unique experiences. I was glad when we had a trip planned or big concert or another event to attend. Otherwise, the day-to-day routine seemed never-ending. Mike's death brought a unique experience, though not a desirable one. There was so much to do afterwards, so many decisions to evaluate, so many appointments to arrange, so many plans to make. There was nothing routine in the aftermath of death. Yet the idea of returning to a regular life seemed disloyal. Donna Tartt's (2013) character in *Goldfinch* was in the same position when she posited "commonplace happiness was lost when I lost her."

And I found I craved the routine, the mundane. In the movie *Yesterday*, Jack says, "Things can get back to normal. And isn't normal wonderful!" I wished for nothing more than for Mike to come home at six o'clock to dinner on the table. For us to share our day while we ate, and then him to put away the food while I cleared the dishes. We would then sit on the recliners with a hot cup of tea each and relax to *Wheel of Fortune*. That was not my reality anymore. "When you have grown accustomed to orbiting every day around someone whose company you enjoy and have grown to depend on—and suddenly that person is gone—your minute-by-minute existence is thrown into disarray" (Wolfelt 2016).

Ricky Gervais, when talking about the main character in his TV series, *After Life*, confides that after the character's partner dies, he finds "He needs to walk the dog; it keeps him alive." He adds that the time after a death "makes you appreciate the mundane things in life . . . those things can save you."

A speech by US Navy Admiral William H. McRaven (2014) starts with, "If you want to change the world, start off by making your bed." Creating order, like making a bed, can help to eliminate one place of chaos in a life. I hadn't heard this speech when I realized this. But I knew I needed a sense of order after this upheaval in my life. So, I started making my bed. I had never made my bed in the past. It gave me a small, granted, but tangible feeling of control and order in my day. Every day.

Things that are mundane or routine give a sense of security. It makes us feel safe to know that all will occur again the same way and we will know how to respond again in the same way. It provides a reassuring constant in our lives.

All that is to say that losing the regular clockwork of a regular day took away my sense of security and safety. Not that I was vulnerable, but that I became wary of making any decisions, afraid to make a mistake. I wanted to honour Mike's memory and value what I had and was now. But I felt so much pressure with this responsibility. I probably overdid it. Everything became a possible memorial!

BEFORE AND AFTER

Another learning I will forever take from this experience is the meaningful reality of before and after. So many things in my conversation and activity are divided into before Mike died and *after* he was gone. It will be a hard stop in the timeline of my life and memories.

One of the things I now have in common with those who have lost loved ones is the knowledge of what grief and loss feels like. Although the circumstances are different for each one, loss teaches us all great lessons. One of those lessons is how to comfort others who have lost someone. Just the fact that we are part of the same club of grievers can bring comfort. Knowing what isn't helpful is comforting. Comfort may be sitting beside someone. It may be bringing tissue. It may be holding a hand. Or texting a knowing message.

The empathy I feel for those experiencing loss in every tragedy is overwhelming. Wisdom from 2 Corinthians 1:4 says that we receive comfort so that we can comfort those in any trouble with the comfort we ourselves receive (BibleGateway.com). This suggests a rationale for the empathy I feel. One of the additional difficult parts of this journey is that since Mike, each family in our Tofino family has lost a loved one. I have tried to support and comfort the families, with the empathy I have and from what I have learned.

The common bond of all the stories I heard, from interviews and smaller anecdotes, was that it is important to feel your grief—to live and express what you feel, when you feel it.

But the flip side of grief is hope. The thing that will keep people going on bad days, and spur them to action on good days, is hope. The hope may be in doing something for others, or in spending time with your other kids or grandkids, or making a difference at your job. But we all need to hope. Hope, in something bigger than yourself, helps make the grieving feel purposeful. It gives continued meaning to our lives. David Kessler (2019) in his book, *Finding Meaning*, calls this the sixth stage of grief. He had written extensively on grief, but after experiencing the tragic loss of his son, searched for more, and found hope through looking for meaning in life.

WHAT I DID TO HELP MYSELF

After three months, I eventually contacted our local hospice society. They put me on the list for the next evening class they were offering. I took the class, glad mostly to have a regularly scheduled thing to do each week. I did my homework and read the assigned book, but didn't find much of it applied to me. So many of the lessons were questions about the future, and I didn't know what mine would look like yet, or even if I would have one. The videos they showed were helpful, and the discussion we had around the group was so valuable. My classmates there became my support group, and then became my friends.

Hospice staff also mentioned a drop-in coffee group that met every Thursday for a couple hours, for people with a recent experience of loss of a loved one. That support group was such a godsend. Those women all became my unlikely friends. That is, in other circumstances I would have nothing in common with most of them, and so would not have connected with them. I knew a couple of the women from the community. But we all had unique experiences of the death of a partner. We helped each other with filling in forms, and through the dreaded "firsts"—first Christmas after, first birthday after, first anniversary after. The support truly became friendship.

MEMORIALS

The funeral home in Scotland crafted a wooden box with a brass plate for Mike's ashes. It sat on a shelf in our den for about four months. My son suggested we scatter some ashes at Moraine Lake, the place where Mike and I had spent our honeymoon, and that he loved dearly. It is a beautiful alpine lake that was featured on the Canadian twenty dollar bill for many years. There are seven huge mountains surrounding a pristine emerald lake, and when we stayed there in 1976, there were only seven cabins and a log lodge.

We planned a trip there in mid-August 2018, but the area was so popular, we couldn't drive all the way up the mountain, and had to take a shuttle, while clutching a baggy full of the ashes. We (me, my oldest son, his wife, and their two kids) walked part way around the lake to find a quiet spot. We settled on one, and my son waded into the water to a depth of about a foot. It would have been a sunny day, but there had been severe fires in the area for many weeks, so the sky was completely obliterated by thick grey smoke. Josh dumped the ashes and watched them sink into a little pile on the bottom of the lake. Just then, the clouds of smoke in the sky parted and a single beam of sunlight shone down from heaven, right onto the ashes! I am not exaggerating! I have photos to prove it! What a magical moment!

Then I sent the others away, and cried as I read the poem [i carry your heart with me(i carry it in] by e.e. cummings. Mike loved poetry, always taking a new book of poetry to share with me on trips we took. This one seemed particularly fitting, because although I was leaving some of him there in the lake, I would carry him forever in my heart for the rest of my life:

i carry your heart with me (i carry it in
my heart) i am never without it (anywhere
i go you go, my dear; and whatever is done
by only me is your doing, my darling)
i fear
no fate (for you are my fate, my sweet) i want
no world (for beautiful you are my world, my true)
and it's you are whatever a moon has always meant
and whatever a sun will always sing is you

here is the deepest secret nobody knows
(here is the root of the root and the bud of the bud
and the sky of the sky of a tree called life; which grows
higher than the soul can hope or mind can hide)
and this is the wonder that's keeping the stars apart

i carry your heart (i carry it in my heart)

One of the women from the support group found a glass blower who would take some ashes and use them with paint to make unique glass objects. So, a number of us trekked there and I had two glass paper weights made with ashes in them (photo in Chapter 5).

The next place we will scatter ashes is into the Vedder River that flows as a tributary of the Fraser River. And the final place we will scatter ashes is the Pacific Ocean, near Tofino, BC. That was our place of bliss. Our place, where we would live if we won the lottery! Again, Mike loved the outdoors and this will mean he is present in river, lake, and ocean.

I, my two sons, daughter-in-law, and oldest grandson agreed to get tattoos of the same Celtic knot image, as a memorial to Mike. My daughter got one later, and my granddaughter said she will when she is older.

On the first anniversary of his death, we went away to Sooke, BC, a little town on the Pacific Ocean. On my way over on the ferry, I found a bracelet with the same line from the e.e. cummings poem on it, so had to buy it! We had most of our Tofino Family join us for an Easter dinner of turkey with all the fixings. It seemed meaningful that it was Easter weekend, traditionally a time celebrating new life. I was prepared to have a toast or some remembrance, but everyone started telling stories of our past times together, and I didn't want to bring down the buoyant atmosphere. Even without it being specifically about Mike, there was a memorial feeling to the weekend.

I participated at the hospice in making a memorial tile with a saying on it. People did various things, some with pictures, some with poems or sayings. I used a line from the e.e. cummings poem, but the tile, alas, was ugly. I threw it out. Not all memorials are worthy!

I still haven't sold Mike's car. I don't drive it. It sits in my garage. It feels like the last thing of value to him; it was a place he spent many hours, and a vehicle he really enjoyed. So, I haven't sold it. There will be a right time for that. But I clearly have more journeying to do.

FOURTEEN MONTHS LATER

I have an amazing job that gives me unbelievable opportunities. I was given the chance to go to Scotland to explore partnerships with fellow universities and colleges. This was good for my department, but this was also so good for me. My colleague that I travelled with is a very sensitive soul, and I trusted her to support me if I needed help in the land where Mike had died.

I had never been to Scotland and didn't know what to expect. I let my colleague, having been there before, plan our itinerary. On days we didn't have meetings, she arranged for some sightseeing. Our first trip was to Loch Lomond. We arrived under a cloudy sky, as most days are there! I had mentioned to Monique, my colleague, that Mike had spent a lot of time at this lake, eating his lunch by the castle and admiring the scenery. I also said I might want some alone time there. I said I would find a quiet place to be by myself by the waterfront, and reflect on being in a place Mike had treasured. Monique went paddle-boarding to give me space. Mike had texted me from there, sharing about the castle, the lake, and the lunch he was enjoying on the hill.

As I sat on a bench, I marveled that I didn't feel anything. No sadness, no longing, nothing. I played a couple of the Scottish songs we had played at the funeral service—*I'll Take the High Road* and *Scotland the Brave*—still nothing. Then, literally out of the blue, an air ambulance helicopter flew low overhead and landed nearby. I soon heard the "wee-wa, wee-wa" siren of a ground ambulance. Without thinking, I stood and started running toward the helicopter. I felt I should help. But what could I do? I stopped where I was and thought . . . there would already be a doctor on the helicopter and equipment and support people in the ambulance. Mike had been attended by a doctor who was helicoptered in within ten minutes of his collapse. An ambulance also came to The Way for him. I couldn't help this person, and I couldn't have helped Mike.

All at once I started blubbering. Big tears, with big guttural sobs. I couldn't catch my breath for all the crying and started gasping for air. And just as if heaven felt my pain, it started raining, big splashy droplets of rain.

I finally realized the burden I had carried! I had felt guilty about not being there to help Mike. I wouldn't have been on the trail with him anyway, but I still felt bad that I didn't help him in any way when he died. So many well-meaning people had asked me, "Were you there with him?" and over and over I had to say no. "Well, did you go over there after he died?" Again, no. I had been carrying this huge amount of guilt and pain on my shoulders. Those raindrops, mixed with my tears, washed away that pain. I no longer had to feel guilty about not being with him when he died.

And just as I recognized this huge relief, my colleague appeared, having heard the helicopter too, wondering if I would need support. She is a person of true empathy.

Near the roadway, at the entrance to the lake area, there was a place to donate to the Scottish Land Commission. I thought it would be fitting to do this, in Mike's name, one of many ways I have found to honour him and keep his memory alive. In his few days there, he had shared with me how he loved the land so much. The Scottish Land Commission wrote me later, saying that the donation qualified me to be a landowner in Scotland, and as such, receive the title of Lady of Glencoe, after a small town. Glencoe, as it turned out, was a town closest to where he died. So, though I gave the donation for him, I felt I received something very precious myself.

The next long journey we did, on another cloudy day, was a tour of the West Highland Way by van. At some point our guide had asked, and I had told him that my partner had died on The Way the previous year. He then was so kind to point out hikers along the path as we drove by. He showed meaningful places, and then asked if I knew where Mike was when he died. I described the scene from pictures Mike had taken. The guide took us to the spot and said, "You need to walk on The Way". He took me by the hand and we walked down to the trail. It was a surreal experience. I felt rooted in the spot. I stood and took it all in, taking photos in every direction, knowing that I was seeing what Mike had seen in his last minutes of life. And just then, again heaven opened a little, but this time with a strong beam of sunshine right onto the trail on the hill ahead of me, possibly where he died. The guide said that that never happens, as it is so rarely sunny there. It made me smile. It was reminiscent of the moment when we sprinkled his ashes in Moraine Lake.

I checked Mike's camera when I returned home, and there was a time-stamped photo he had taken ten minutes before he died, of the exact place on The Way where I had walked.

MY POSTHUMOUS BIRTHDAY GIFT

My 60th birthday was to be three weeks after Mike returned from Scotland. He had planned an elegant dinner party for twenty with great detail, including a string quartet, outdoor tenting and heaters, a caterer, and a dance instructor to construct a sort of *Dancing with the Stars* experience. This was an homage to our ballroom dance lessons.

He told me about the plans, as he knew I didn't like surprises. He consulted with me on the songs I wanted for the dancing (*Shut Up and Dance* by Walk the Moon, and *Thinking Out Loud* by Ed Sheeran), and he added *Perfect* by Ed Sheeran, just for him and me ("We were just kids when we fell in love . . . I found a woman stronger than anyone I know . . ."). That will forever be our song (along with *Brown Eyed Girl* by Van Morrison, our original "our song"), after dancing to it in our living room so many evenings. I had to go through all his notes and undo his reservations and orders, as I couldn't have the party. It would have been five days after his funeral! What a sweet memory of how he wanted to celebrate me!

One of the things that wasn't in his notebook was anything about a diamond ring. We had looked at three different ones to commemorate my birthday, but had not decided anything. He had privately asked the jeweler to bring all the rings in and then to hold them until my party. A few days after my birthday I received a call from the jewelry store asking if I still wanted the rings. I was shocked. I wanted one, but didn't know if I should still get it. My kids convinced me to choose a ring as a wearable memory of his romantic side. The salesperson said Mike told her he liked the one with rose gold and yellow gold because it was "two-toned, just like us" (L. Abraham, personal communication, May 13, 2018).

AND NOW

As I write this, it is almost two years since Mike died. I can't believe it's been that long. I still miss him. I still love him. I wish he was still here. Dating has been fraught with challenges, as no new man seems to measure up to what I had with Mike. It is especially poignant as we plan my daughter's wedding, and he is not here to give her away in the ceremony.

But, I have moved to a place of peace and contentment and independence. I am living alone for the first time in my life, and enjoying it! There will be more learning and growth, no doubt, as I anticipate that this journey of grief will continue in some form for my whole life.

Going anywhere with Mike was an adventure, given his propensity to try things in unorthodox ways. After he died, I found a T-shirt based on the Disney movie *Up*, that says, "He was my greatest adventure." It is so fitting.

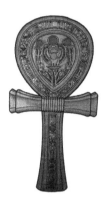

Chapter 4

Mind Map of the Journey of Grief & Loss

> "We all lose those we love and this
> is a great unifying trust amongst humans."
> *Shilpi Somay Gowda, author of The Shape of Family*

MIND MAP OF THE JOURNEY OF LOSS DUE TO DEATH

SUDDEN DEATH

- No chance to say goodbye
- Greater chance of denial
- Regret of things unsaid or undone
- No way to know loved one's wishes
- No way to know what memorial arrangements to make
- No chance to plan
- Added issues if there were "other" people (disenfranchised grief)

DEATH

DEATH BY LIFE LIMITING ILLNESS

- Due to illness
- Exhausting
- Anticipatory grief
- Lots of anger and bargaining
- Chance to discuss memorial plans
- Chance to give away items to family
- Guilt of relief when loved one dies
- The death is expected but still a shock

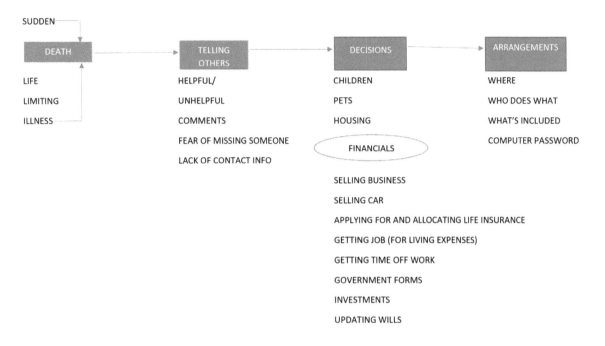

SUDDEN

DEATH

LIFE

LIMITING

ILLNESS

TELLING OTHERS

HELPFUL/

UNHELPFUL

COMMENTS

FEAR OF MISSING SOMEONE

LACK OF CONTACT INFO

DECISIONS

CHILDREN

PETS

HOUSING

FINANCIALS

SELLING BUSINESS

SELLING CAR

APPLYING FOR AND ALLOCATING LIFE INSURANCE

GETTING JOB (FOR LIVING EXPENSES)

GETTING TIME OFF WORK

GOVERNMENT FORMS

INVESTMENTS

UPDATING WILLS

ARRANGEMENTS

WHERE

WHO DOES WHAT

WHAT'S INCLUDED

COMPUTER PASSWORD

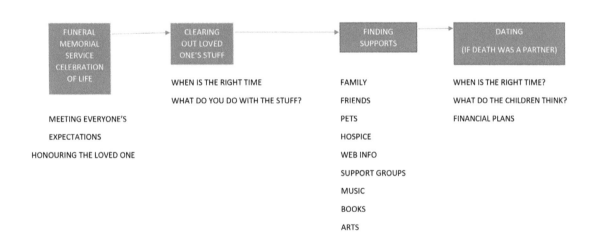

FUNERAL MEMORIAL SERVICE CELEBRATION OF LIFE

MEETING EVERYONE'S

EXPECTATIONS

HONOURING THE LOVED ONE

CLEARING OUT LOVED ONE'S STUFF

WHEN IS THE RIGHT TIME

WHAT DO YOU DO WITH THE STUFF?

FINDING SUPPORTS

FAMILY

FRIENDS

PETS

HOSPICE

WEB INFO

SUPPORT GROUPS

MUSIC

BOOKS

ARTS

DATING (IF DEATH WAS A PARTNER)

WHEN IS THE RIGHT TIME?

WHAT DO THE CHILDREN THINK?

FINANCIAL PLANS

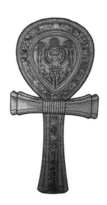

Chapter 5

. . . .

Photos of Memorials

"Everything leaves eventually in the physical form, but the
memories of good people and good work are timeless."
Jimmy Buffet, singer, composer, author

When we lose the physical being of a loved one, many of us are emotionally challenged to find a way to keep his or her memory alive. Some memorialize their loved one with a headstone in a cemetery. Others keep an urn of cremated remains. There are many ways to keep the memory of your loved one present. The photos below are examples of what some have done to provide a legacy:

ANCIENT EGYPT

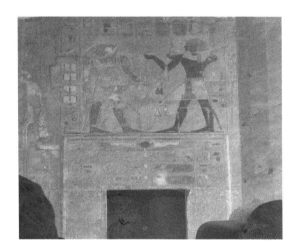

This masoleum has hieroglyphic inscriptions of the exploits of the pharaoh buried here.

The magnificent temple at Luxor was built by Amenhotep III, Ramses II, and completed by Tutankhamun.

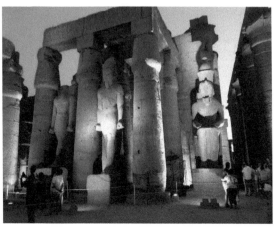

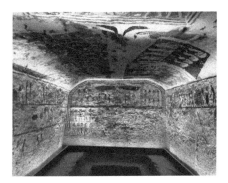

This is a tomb in the Valley of the Kings.

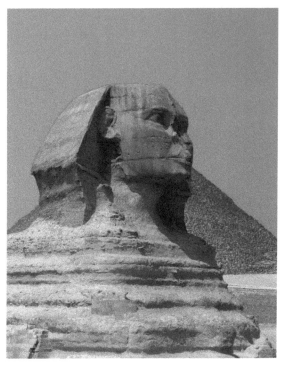

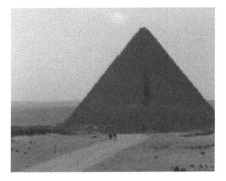

The Great Sphinx is thought to have had the celestial purpose to resurrect the soul of Pharaoh Khafre by channeling the power of the sun and other gods.

This is one of the pyramids of Giza, constructed as a burial chamber for a pharaoh.

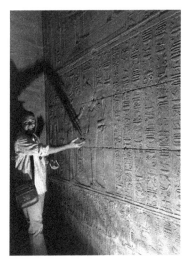

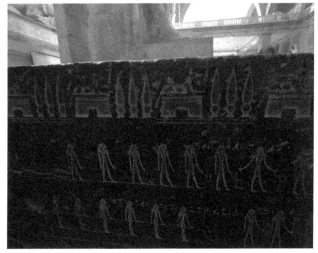

The ankh symbol of life (literally breath of life) was sculpted everywhere in the tombs of kings, to signify their belief in the afterlife. Other hieroglyph depictions included the food, animals, and servants that were buried alive to aid the king in his journey to heaven.

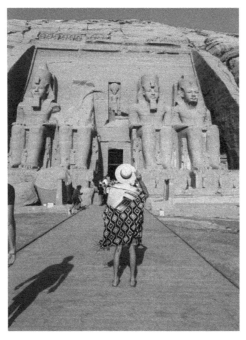

The miracle of engineering was apparent in this temple in Abu Simbel, where, with no windows or source of natural light, a statue of the pharaoh Ramses as a god, set far back in this monument, was illuminated by the sun.

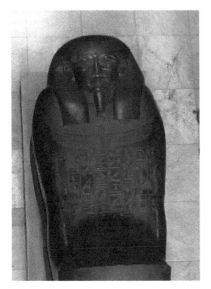

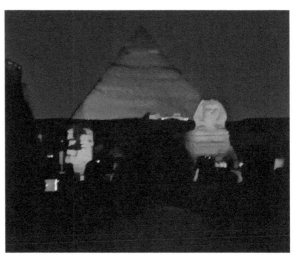

Outside of Cairo, this shows a pyramid and the Sphinx illuminated at night.

This is a well-preserved sarcophagus.

NEW ORLEANS JAZZ FUNERAL AND GHOSTLY HISTORY

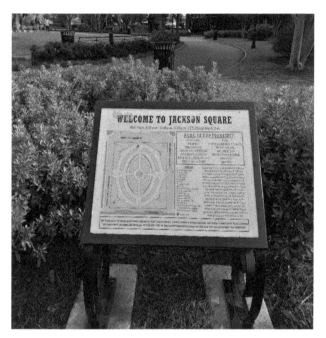 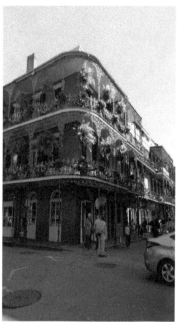

Jackson Square is a National Historic Landmark in the centre of New Orleans, commemorating the lives and deaths from early battle., It has significance in some of the ghost history of the area, and is now an area for street performers and shopping.

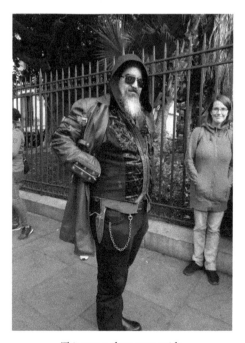

This was a ghost tour guide.

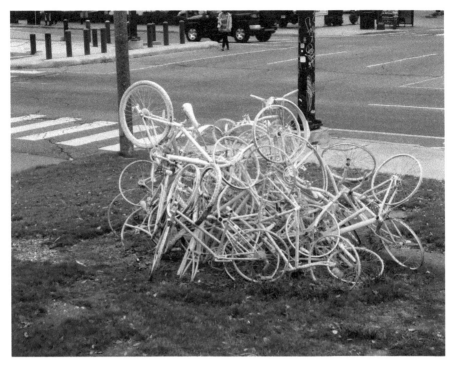

The city is relatively flat so is conducive to bike transportation. This sculpture was erected as a memorial to pay respect to a bike courier who was killed in a collision with a truck.

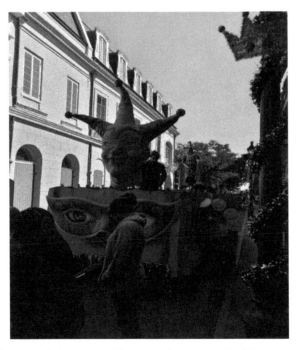

These Mardi Gras floats were being prepared for a scene in a movie. Mardi Gras is an event signifying the beginning of the Catholic tradition of Lent, leading up to the celebration of the resurrection at Easter.

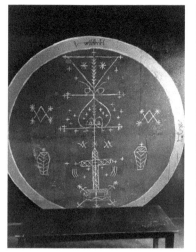 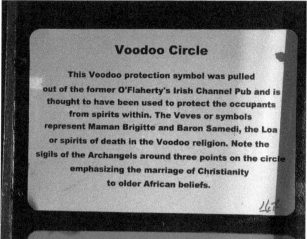

Voodoo is a combination of African traditions brought by slaves and the Christian traditions introduced to slaves by their masters.

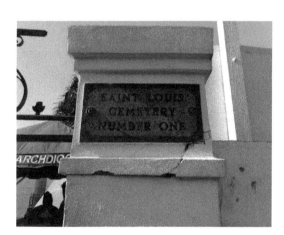

Cemetery Number One is the most famous of the cemeteries and has been the site of ghostly activity as well as vandalism. No one is allowed on the property without a guide.

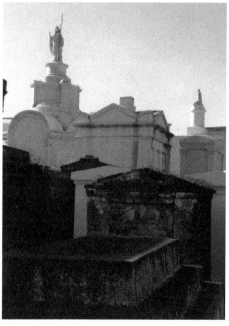

Graves are above ground as the city itself exists below sea level.

MIKE

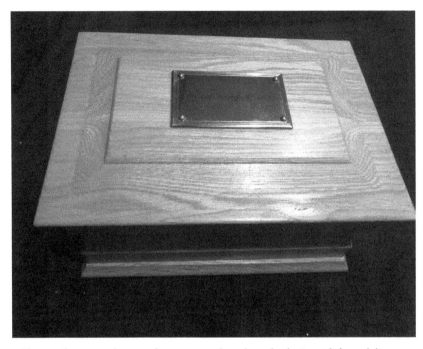

This wooden urn with name plaque was made and sent by the Scottish funeral director.

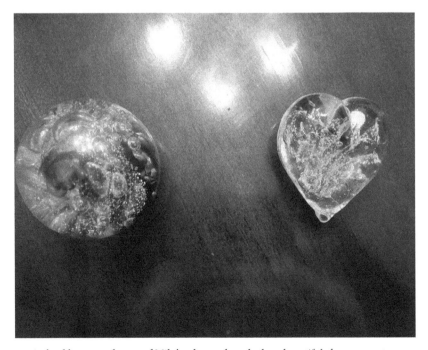

A glassblower used some of Mike's ashes and made these beautiful glass mementoes.

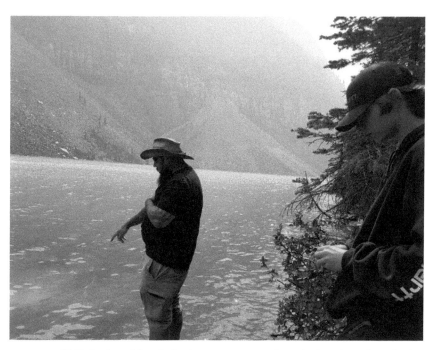

When we scattered Mike's ashes, although the sky was overcast with smoke from forest fires, the sky opened and a small sunbeam shone down directly onto the place where the ashes were laid.

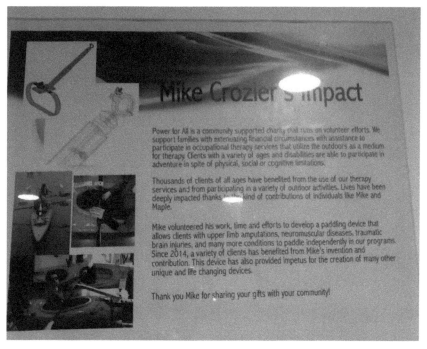

Power for All Society received Mike's engineering support in his life and donations in his death; they offered this tribute for his help.

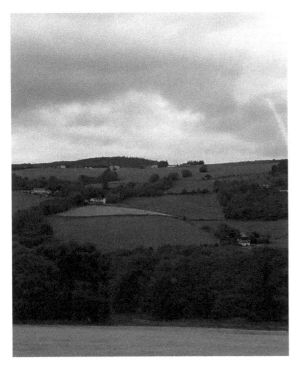
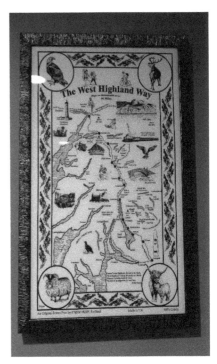

These are some of the beautiful hills where Mike spent his
last days while walking the West Highland Way trail.

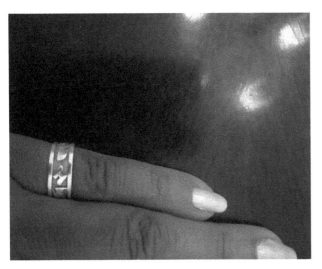
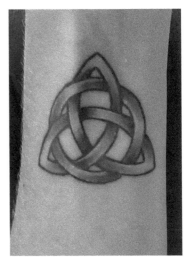

A silversmith in Egypt made this ring with the hieroglyph lettering
of Mike's name.

The immediate family got tattoos
of this Celtic knot as a permanent
remembrance of Mike's Irish heritage.

OTHER MEMORIALS

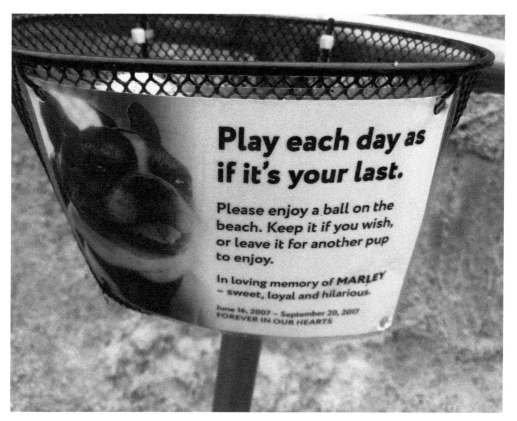

This sign was on a beach in Santa Cruz, California.

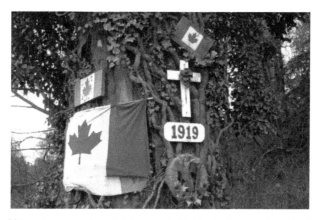

This tree is a World War I memorial created by Charlie Perkins in 1919 for his friends who didn't make it home. When the freeway was being put through this area, Perkins protested the removal of this tree, so the engineers adjusted the design so the road curved around the tree. Everyone who drives Highway 1 near Vancouver saw this memorial, until the tree itself died.

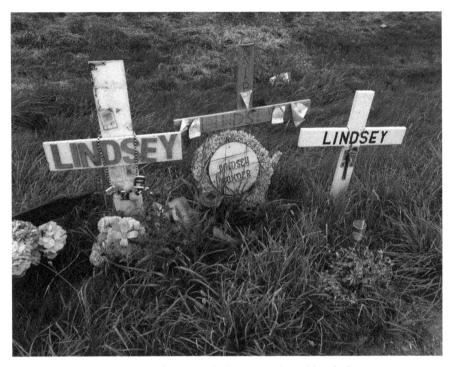

This is one of many roadside memorials in Abbotsford.

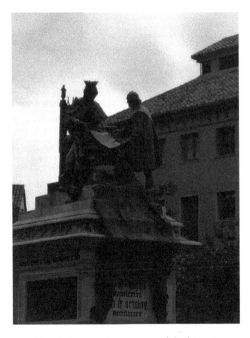

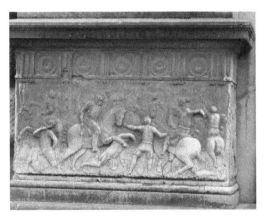

Friezes such as this are sculpted onto the palace and fortress in Alhambra, Spain commemorating famous battles.

This statue was in memory of the historic arrangement between Queen Isabella and Christopher Columbus.

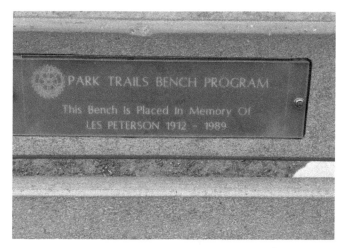

Many people purchase benches along rivers or in parks to memorialize their loved ones, human or pet, and give something back to their community.

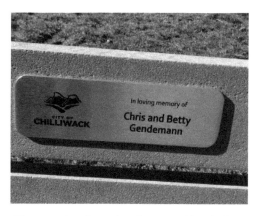

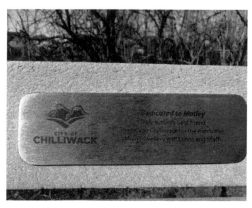

This is a privately purchased memorial bench along a public trail

This bench is how some people memorialize their pet.

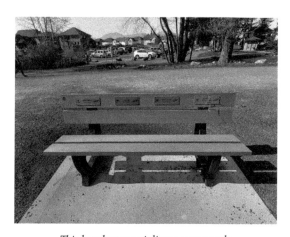

This bench memorializes many people

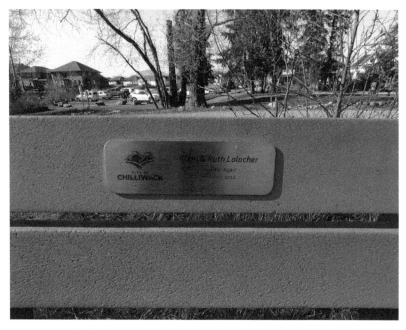

This bench is how some people memorialize their loved ones.

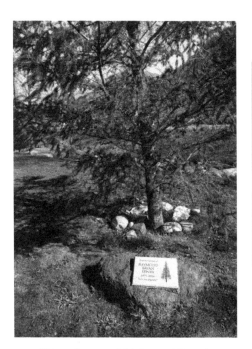

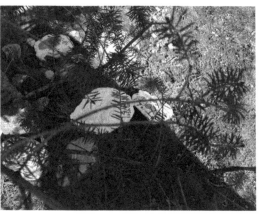

Another loved one remembered with painted rocks.

This rock memorial is in a public park.

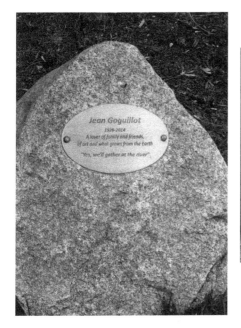

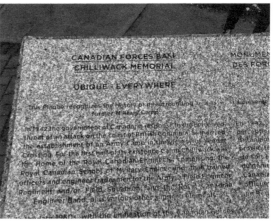

These is part of a mass memorial on a Canadian
Forces Base.

This rock memorial is by the Vedder River

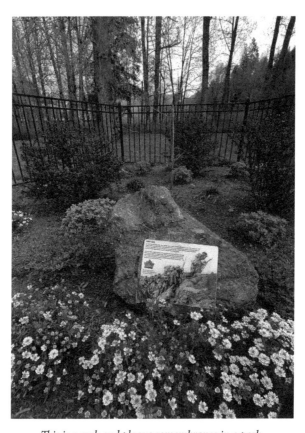

This is a rock and plaque remembrance in a park.

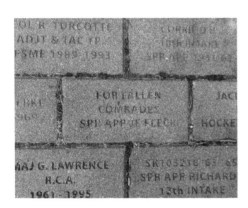

Some of the many Canadian Forces members memorialized on the Chilliwack Base

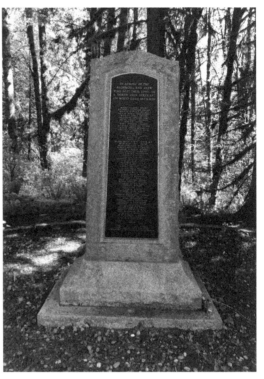

This is a tribute to the passengers and crew who lost their lives from a Northstar Aircraft crash on Mt. Slesse.

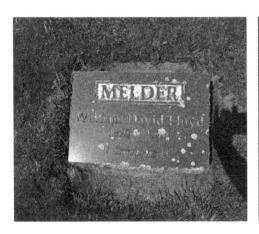

A traditional memorial in Western culture is the gravestone: this one for my dad.

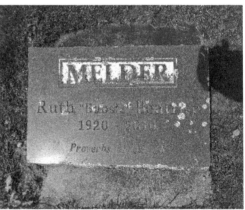

This gravestone is for my mom.

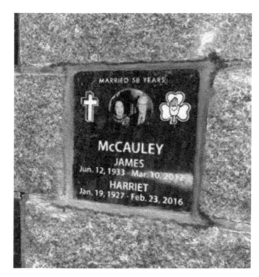

This grave marker is for a friend's parents.

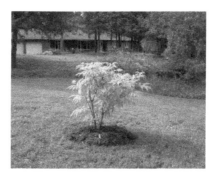

This tree was planted for Reid who died in a car accident.
His mom placed some of his ashes at the base when she planted the tree,
so life could come from his loss.

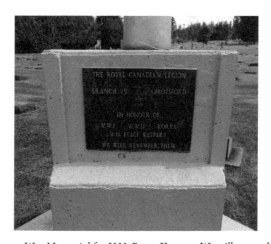

This is a Korean War Memorial for U.N. Peace Keepers. We will remember them all.

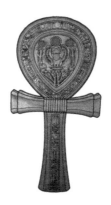

Resources

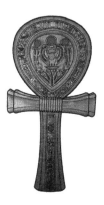

Supportive Music

"Music is no more than the sound of our regrets
put to a cadence that stirs the illusion of hope."

Andre Acuman, author

Music is a form of art that speaks to the human soul. Songs affect us emotionally. Hearing one of "our" songs on the radio, or a sad song about loss caused me to have to pull over my car and cry by the side of the road. I sought out the feeling of sadness, at times, to help me strongly feel the pain rather than numbness. I took comfort in it. I found healing in the messages these musical artists had written, seeming to understand what I had been through. Along with some that were suggested by websites, and others by friends, here are some of the songs I would play while I sat and cried for hours:

SONGS ABOUT SORROW, GRIEF, AND LOST LOVED ONES

Updated on June 15, 2020
Non-exhaustive, non-curated

	TITLE	ARTIST
1.	Address in the Stars	Caitlin & Will
2.	Almost Home	Moby
3.	A Long December	Counting Crows
4.	And I Love Her	Beatles
5.	A Picture of Me (Without You)	Lorrie Morgan
6.	Angel	The Corrs
7.	Angel Flying Too Close to the Ground	Willie Nelson
8.	A Song for Mama	Boyz to Men
9.	The Baby	Blake Shelton
10.	Being with You	Smokey Robinson
11.	Better Together	Jack Johnson
12.	Birds	Imagine Dragons
13.	Blackbird	Alter Bridge
14.	Blue Eyes Crying in the Rain	Willie Nelson
15.	Bridge Over Troubled Water	Simon & Garfunkel

16.	Bye Bye	Mariah Carey
17.	Can't Get Enough of your Love Baby	Barry White
18.	Can You See Me	Krista Siegfrids
19.	The Car	Jeff Carson
20.	Closer to the Light	Bruce Cockburn
21.	Clouds	Before You Exit
22.	Cold	Jeff Williams
23.	Crash	Sum41
24.	Cryin' for Me (Wayman's Song)	Toby Keith
25.	The Dance	Garth Brooks
26.	Dancing in the Sky	Dani and Lizzy
27.	Dance with My Father	Luther Vandross
28.	Don't Take the Girl	Tim McGraw
29.	Drink a Beer	Luke Bryan
30.	Edge of Glory	Lady Gaga
31.	El Paso	Marty Robbins
32.	Emma	Hot Chocolate
33.	Even in Death	Evanesence
34.	Everybody Hurts	REM
35.	Everybody Lost Somebody	Bleachers
36.	Fade In/Fade Out	Nothing More
37.	Father, You Believed	Catman Cohen
38.	Fire and Rain	James Taylor
39.	Fly	Celine Dion
40.	Forever	Rascal Flatts
41.	Forever & Always	Dylan Matthew
42.	Free Bird	Lynyrd Skyryrd
43.	Gone Away	The Offspring
44.	Gone Too Soon	Michael Jackson
45.	Gone Too Soon	Daughtry
46.	Gone Too Soon	Simple Plan
47.	Goodbye My Friend	Keali'i Riechel
48.	Goodbye my friend	by Linda Rondstat

49.	Go Rest High on That Mountain	Vince Gill
50.	Grace	Kate Havneveik
51.	The Greatest Man I Never Knew	Reba McEntire
52.	Go Rest High on That Mountain	Vince Gill
53.	Hard Habit to Break	Chicago
54.	Have I Told You Lately That I Love You	Rod Stewart
55.	Hear You Me	Jimmy Eats World
56.	Heaven	Beyonce
57.	Heaven Got Another Angel	Gordon Garner
58.	Heaven Was Needing a Hero	Jo Dee Messina
59.	Hello	Adele
60.	Here Today	Paul McCartney
61.	He's My Son	Mark Schultz
62.	He Stopped Loving Her Today	George Jones
63.	Holes in the Floor of Heaven	Steve Wariner
64.	Hold On	Wilson Phillips
65.	Hold On	Chord Overstreet
66.	Home	Jeff Williams (featuring Casey Lee Williams)
67.	Homesick	MercyMe
68.	Honey (I Miss You)	Bobby Goldsboro
69.	How Can I Help You Say Goodbye	Patty Loveless
70.	How Could You Leave Us?	NF
71.	How Do I Live Without You	Leanne Rhimes
72.	How Do You Sleep	Sam Smith
73.	Hurt	Christina Aguilera
74.	I Cross My Heart	George Strait
75.	I Drive Your Truck	Lee Brice
76.	If I Die Young	The Band Perry
77.	If Heaven Had a Face	Joe Jury
78.	If I Get High Enough	Nothing but Thieves
79.	If I Had Only Known	Reba McEntire
80.	If I Have To Go	Tom Waits

81.	If the World Was Ending	JP Saxe
82.	If Today Was Your Last Day	Nickleback
83.	If You Came Back From Heaven	Lorrie Morgan
84.	If You Could See Me Fly	Annie Morgan
85.	If You Could See Me Now	The Script
86.	If You're Reading This	Tim McGraw
87.	I Grieve	Peter Gabriel
88.	I Lived	OneRepublic
89.	I'll Be Missing You	Puff Daddy featuring Faith Evans
90.	I'll See You Again	Westlife
91.	I'll Wait for You	Joe Nichols
92.	I Miss My Friend	Darryl Worrley
93.	I Miss you a little	John Michael Montgomery
94.	I'm Not Gonna Miss You	Glen Campbell and The Wrecking Crew
95.	Impossible	Shontelle
96.	I'm Sorry	John Denver
97.	In Loving Memory	Alter Bridge
98.	In My Dreams	James Morrison
99.	In My Life (I Love You More)	The Beatles
100.	In the Arms of an Angel	Sarah McLachlan
101.	Into the Light	In This Moment
102.	Into the West	Annie Lennox
103.	I Pray	Amanda Perez
104.	I Promise It's Not Goodbye	Chris Cornell
105.	I remember L.A.	Celine Dion;
106.	Is that All There is?	Peggy Lee
107.	I Still Miss You	Keith Anderson
108.	It's So Hard to Say Goodbye to Yesterday"	Boyz II Men
109.	Jealous of the Angels	Donna Taggart
110.	Joanne	Lady Gaga
111.	Just a dream	Carrie Underwood
112.	Just Like Them Horses	Reba McEntire

113.	King of Sorrow	Sade
114.	Kiss From a Rose	Sea
115.	Last Kiss	Pearl Jam
116.	Lay Me Down	Sam Smith
117.	Leave Out All the Rest	Linkin Park
118.	Let Her Go	Passenger
119.	Let It Be	The Beatles
120.	Life Without You	Stevie Ray Vaughan
121.	Like I'm Gonna Lose you	Meghan Trainor and John Legend
122.	Like Jesus to a Child	George Michaels
123.	Little Soldier	Trey Healy
124.	Live Like You Were Dying	Tim McGraw
125.	Looking for an Answer	Mike Shinoda/Linkin Park
126.	Lose You to Love Me	Selena Gomez
127.	Love is a Verb	John Mayer
128.	Love Is Stronger Than Death	Angela McCluskey
129.	Love Letters	Ketty Lester
130.	Love Me	Collin Raye
131.	Love takes time	Mariah Carey
132.	Lucy	Skillet
133.	Memories	Maroon 5
134.	Miss Emily's Picture	John Conlee
135.	My Angel	Kellie Pickler
136.	My Father's Eyes	Eric Clapton
137.	My Heart Will Go On"	Celine Dion
138.	My Immortal	Evanescence
139.	My Son	Gary Puckett & The Union Gap
140.	Nightingale	Demi Lovato
141.	Nobody Knows It But Me	Tony Rich Project
142.	Not a Day Goes By	Lonestar
143.	Objects in the rearview mirror may appear closer than they are	Meatloaf
144.	One Hell of an Amen	Brantley Gilbert

145.	One More Day	Diamond Rio
146.	One More Light	Linkin Park
147.	Only the Good Die Young	Billy Joel
148.	Ordinary World	Duran Duran
149.	Over You	Miranda Lambert
150.	Panama	Quinn XCII
151.	Perfect	Ed Sheeran
152.	Photograph	Ed Sheeran
153.	Picture Perfect	Escape the Fate
154.	Please Remember	LeAnn Rimes
155.	Probably Wouldn't Be This Way	LeAnn Rimes
156.	Promise to Try	Madonna
157.	Radios in Heaven	Plain White T's
158.	Red Rag Top	Tim McGraw
159.	Rocky	Austin Roberts
160.	Ronan	Taylor Swift
161.	Roses for the Dead	Funeral for a Friend
162.	Safe & Sound	Taylor Swift
163.	Saturn	Sleeping at Last
164.	See You Again	Carrie Underwood
165.	See You Again	Charlie Puth
166.	See You On the Other Side	Ozzy Osbourne
167.	Shadow of the Day	Linkin Park
168.	Shallow	Lady Gaga
169.	She's Gone	Hall & Oates
170.	Sinner	Andy Grammer
171.	Sissy's Song	Alan Jackson
172.	Slipped Away	Avril Lavigne
173.	Small Bump	Ed Sheeran
174.	So Far Away	Avenged Sevenfold
175.	Someone Like You	Adele
176.	Someone You Loved	Lewis Capaldi
177.	Supermarket Flowers	Ed Sheeran

178.	Tears in Heaven	Eric Clapton
179.	Temporary Home	Carrie Underwood
180.	There You'll Be	Faith Hill
181.	This Is Your Song	Ronan Keating
182.	Together Again	Janet Jackson
183.	To Where You Are	Josh Groban
184.	Travelin' Soldier	Dixie Chicks
185.	The Truth	Jason Aldean.
186.	Unchained Melody	Righteous Brothers
187.	Waiting on Sunshine	Amy Rose
188.	Wake Me Up When September Ends	Green Day
189.	Walk of life by	Walk of life by
190.	We're Gonna Ride Again	Brantley Gilbert
191.	What hurts the most	Rascal Flatts;
192.	When I Get Where I'm Going	Brad Paisley
193.	When I'm Gone	Joey + Rory
194.	Wherever You Will You	The Calling
195.	Where Were You (When the World Stopped Turning)	Alan Jackson
196.	Who Knew	Pink
197.	Why	Andra
198.	Why	Rascal Flatts
199.	Will the Circle Be Unbroken	Nitty Gritty Dirt Band
200.	The Wind	Mariah Carey
201.	Wish You Were Here	Incubus
202.	Wish You Were Here	Mark Wills
203.	Without Me	Halsey
204.	Whiskey lullaby	Allison Krause and Brad Paisley
205.	Who You'd Be Today	Kenny Chesney
206.	You Have Been Loved	George Michael
207.	You Look Wonderful Tonight	Eric Clapton
208.	You're Still Here	Faith Hill
209.	You're Still the One	Shania Twain

210.	You Said You'd Grow Old with Me	Michael Schulte
211.	You Should Be Here	Cole Swindell
212.	You Were Loved	Whitney Houston

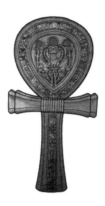

Movies

"When grief is deepest, words are fewest."

Ann Voskamp, Canadian author

Another artistic medium for healing is television and film content. It depicts scenes that we may have lived through, but wouldn't wish on anyone! Television and films reflect real life and let us feel a common bond with others. They demonstrate that we are not alone in our grief.

MOVIES

1000 Acres

A Man Called Ove

A Monster Calls

Amour

A Walk to Remember

Beetlejuice

Beginners

Big Fish

Bonneville

Brian's Song

Bridge to Terabithia

The Bucket List

Camino

Charlie St. Cloud

Citizen Kane

City of Angels

Collateral Beauty

Cries and Whispers

Death at a Funeral

Defending Your Life

Delicacy

Departures

Descendants

The Face of Love

Faces of Death

The Fault In Our Stars

Final Destination

Five People You Meet In Heaven

Flatliners

Ghost

The Grey

Harold and Maude

Hereafter

Lorenzo's Oil

Love Happens

The Lovely Bones

Love Story

Manchester by the Sea

Marvin's Room

Me and Earl and the Dying Girl

Meet Joe Black

Message in a Bottle

Million Dollar Baby

Mully

My Girl

My Life Without Me

My Sister's Keeper

Mystic River

Ordinary People

Philomena

P.S. I Love You

The Rabbit Hole

The Sea Inside

The Secret Life of Bees

The Seventh Seal

The Shack

Silent Heart

Sixth Sense

Sophie's Choice

Stand By Me

Sunset in Heaven

Sweet November

Taking Chance

Tapas

Tea with Mussolini

Tender Mercies

The Rest of Us

Things We Lost in the Fire

This Is Where I Leave You

To Gillian on her 37th Birthday

To Love

Tuesdays with Morrie

Újratervezés

Up

What Dreams May Come

The Wife

Wit

Y Tu Mamá También

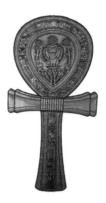

Books, Articles, & Poems

"An examined death is as important as an examined life."

Julia Samuel, author

The written word in books, articles, and poems are repositories of the wisdom of our culture. They store the tales of life and death. Many of the titles listed below are guides, some are personal journeys, and others are support resources. All can be helpful, if the reader finds them applicable:

BOOKS

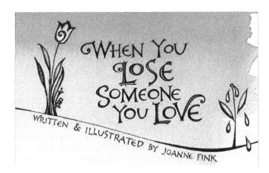

When You Lose someone You Love, by Fink, 2017

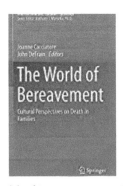

The World of Bereavement: Cultural Perspectives on Death in Families, by Cacciatore and DeFrain, 2015

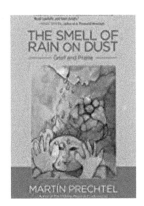

The Smell of Rain on Dust: Grief and Praise, by Prechtel, 2015

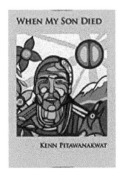

When My Son Died, by Pitawanakwat, 2015

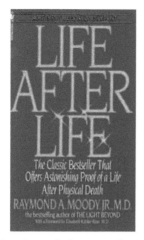

Life After Life, by Moody, 2015

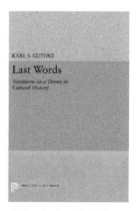

Last Words, by Guthke, 1992

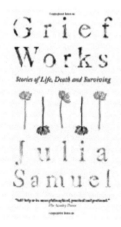

Grief Works, by Samuel, 2018

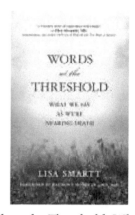

Words at the Threshold: What We
Say as We're Nearing Death,
by Smartt, 2017
This linguist recorded and analyzed the last
words of her dying father, then researched
the last words of many others to see patterns
of metaphors.

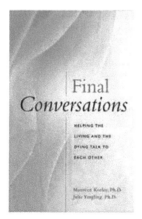

Final Conversation,
by Keeley and Yingling, 2007

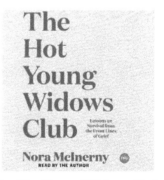

The Hot Young Widows Club,
by McInerny, 2019

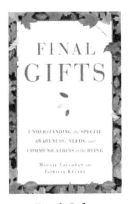

Final Gifts,
by Callanan & Kelley, 2021

Written by two hospice nurses, the book is
the unique communications our dying loved
ones share with us, the survivors, in their
dying. This book has become a touchstone
for caregivers of the terminally ill and dying.

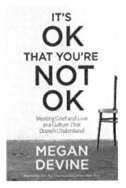

It's OK that you're not OK:
Meeting Grief and Loss in a Culture
That Doesn't Understand,
by Devine & Nepo, 2017

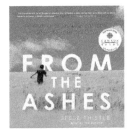

From the Ashes, by Thistle, 2019
"My story of being Metis, homeless, and
finding my way."

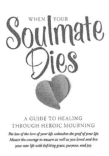

When Your Soulmate Dies,
by Wolfelt, 2016

Find many other books that complement
this title at centreforloss.com.

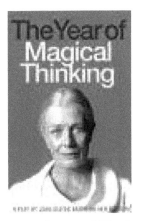

The Year of Magical Thinking,
by Didion, 2007

Talking to Strangers,
by Gladwell, 2019

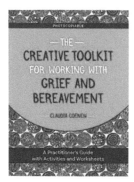

The Creative Toolkit for Working
with Grief and Bereavement:
A Practitioner's Guide with
Activities and Worksheets.
by Coenen & Pimas, 2020

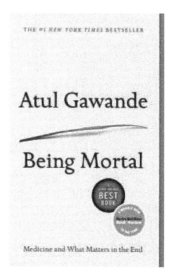

Being Mortal, by Gawande, 2017

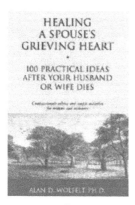

Healing a Spouse's Grieving Heart,
by Wolfelt, 2003

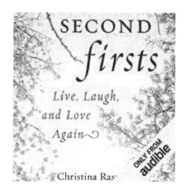

Second Firsts: Live, Laugh, and Love
Again, by Rasmussen, 2013

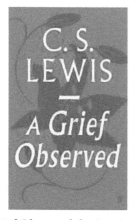

A Grief Observed, by Lewis, 2015

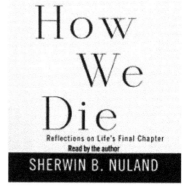

How We Die: Reflections on Life's
Final Chapter, by Nuland, 2008

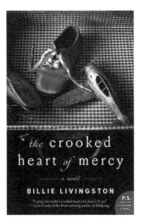

The Crooked Heat of Mercy,
by Livingston, 2016

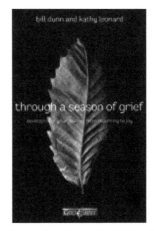

Through a Season of Grief,
by Dunn & Leonard, 2004

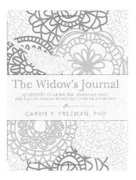

The Widow's Journal: Questions to
Guide You Through Grief and Life
Planning After the Loss of a Partner,
by Freeman, 2015

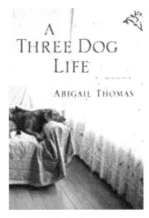

A Three Dog Life, by Thomas, 2007

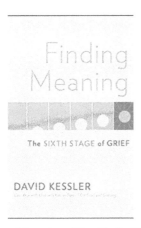

Finding Meaning: The Sixth Stage of
Grief, by Kessler, 2020

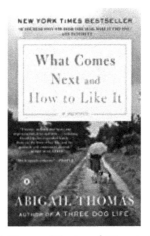

What Comes Next and How to Like
It, by Thomas, 2016

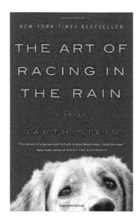

The Art of Racing in the Rain,
by Stein, 2018

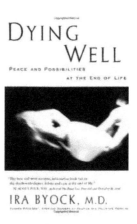

Dying Well, by Byock, 1998

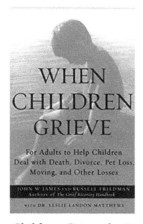

When Children Grieve, by James &
Friedman & Matthews, 2002

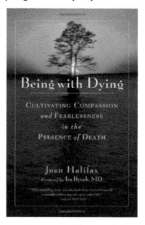

Being with Dying, by Halifax, 2009

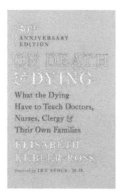

On Death and Dying,
by Kubler Ross, 2014

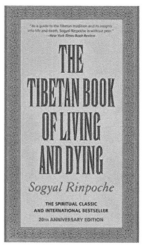

The Tibetan Book of Living and
Dying, by Rinpoche, 2020

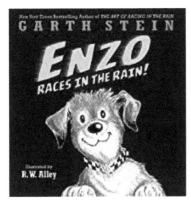

Enzo Races In the Rain,
by Stein, 2014

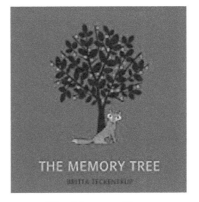

The Memory Tree,
by Teckentrup, 2014

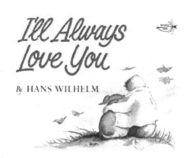

I'll Always Love You,
by Wilhelm, 1988

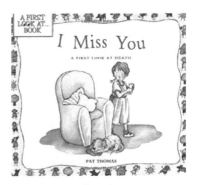

I Miss You, by Thomas, 2001

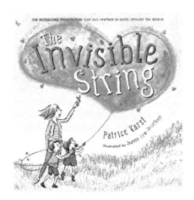

The Invisible String, by Karst, 2018

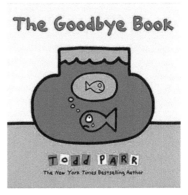

The Goodbye Book, by Parr, 2015

ARTICLES

....

5 Things To Know About Woe, by Becky Ninkovic,
August 24 2019 Vancouver Sun article
Retrieved June 2021 from: https://vancouversun.com/entertainment/
music/5-things-to-know-about-woe-by-becky-ninkovic

The Dinner Party, Like Therapy, But Better by Caitlen Gibson
November 21, 2018 Washington Post article
Retrieved June 2021 from: https://www.washingtonpost.com/lifestyle/style/like-
therapy-but-better-the-holiday-dinner-party-that-makes-space-for-grief/2018/11/20/
fd6626e0-ec63-11e8-8679-934a2b33be52_story.html

POEMS

....

BECAUSE I HAVE LOVED LIFE

Because I have loved life, I shall have no sorrow to die.
I have sent up my gladness on wings, to be lost in the blue of the sky.
I have run and leaped with the rain, I have taken the wind to my breast.
My cheek like a drowsy child to the face of the earth I have pressed.
Because I have loved life, I shall have no sorrow to die.

I have kissed young love on the lips, I have heard his song to the end.
I have struck my hand like a seal in the loyal hand of a friend.
I have known the peace of heaven, the comfort of work done well.
I have longed for death in the darkness and risen alive out of hell.
Because I have loved life, I shall have no sorrow to die.

I give a share of my soul to the world where my course is run.
I know that another shall finish the task I must leave undone.
I know that no flower, nor flint was in vain on the path I trod.
As one looks on a face through a window, through life I have looked on God.
Because I have loved life, I shall have no sorrow to die.

by Amelia Josephine Burr

UNTITLED

And people stayed home
and read books and listened
and rested and exercised
and made art and played
and learned new ways of being
and stopped
and listened deeper

someone meditated
someone prayed

someone danced
someone met their shadow

and people began to think differently
and people healed
and in the absence of people who lived in ignorant ways,
dangerous, meaningless and heartless,
even the earth began to heal

and when the danger ended
and people found each other
grieved for the dead people
and they made new choices
and dreamed of new visions
and created new ways of life
and healed the earth completely
just as they were healed themselves.

by Kitty O'Meara

DEATH IS NOTHING AT ALL

Death is nothing at all.
I have only slipped away to the next room.
I am I and you are you.
Whatever we were to each other,
That, we still are.

Call me by my old familiar name.
Speak to me in the easy way
which you always used.
Put no difference into your tone.
Wear no forced air of solemnity or sorrow.

Laugh as we always laughed
at the little jokes we enjoyed together.
Play, smile, think of me. Pray for me.
Let my name be ever the household word
hat it always was.
Let it be spoken without effect.
Without the trace of a shadow on it.

Life means all that it ever meant.
It is the same that it ever was.
There is absolute unbroken continuity.
Why should I be out of mind
because I am out of sight?

I am but waiting for you.
For an interval.
Somewhere. Very near.
Just around the corner.

All is well.

Nothing is past; nothing is lost. One brief moment and all will be as it was before only better, infinitely happier and forever we will all be one together with Christ.

by Henry Scott Holland

AFTERGLOW

I'd like the memory of me
o be a happy one.
I'd like to leave an afterglow
of smiles when life is done.
I'd like to leave an echo
whispering softly down the ways,
Of happy times and laughing times
and bright and sunny days.
I'd like the tears of those who grieve,
o dry before the sun
of happy memories
hat I leave when life is done.

by Helen Lowrie Marshall

DEATH~WHAT A WONDERFUL WAY TO EXPLAIN IT

A sick man turned to his doctor as he was preparing to leave the examination room and said,
Doctor, I am afraid to die. Tell me what lies on the other side.
Very quietly, the doctor said, I don't know.
You don't know? You're, a Christian man, and don't know what's on the other side?

The doctor was holding the handle of the door; On the other side came a sound of scratching and whining,
and as he opened the door, a dog sprang into the room and leaped on him with an eager show of gladness.
Turning to the patient, the doctor said,

Did you notice my dog? He's never been in this room before.
He didn't know what was inside. He knew nothing except that his master was here,
And when the door opened, he sprang in without fear.
I know little of what is on the other side of death, but I do know one thing...
I know my Master is there and that is enough.

Author Unknown

FAREWELL MY FRIENDS

Farewell My Friends
It was beautiful
As long as it lasted
The journey of my life.
I have no regrets
Whatsoever said
The pain I'll leave behind.
Those dear hearts
Who love and care . . .
And the strings pulling
At the heart and soul . . .
The strong arms
That held me up
When my own strength
Let me down.
At the turning of my life
I came across
Good friends,
Friends who stood by me
Even when time raced me by.
Farewell, farewell My friends
I smile and
Bid you goodbye.
No, shed no tears
For I need them not

All I need is your smile.
If you feel sad
Do think of me
For that's what I'll like
When you live in the hearts
Of those you love
Remember then
You never die.

by Rabindranath Tagore. Also attributed to Gitanjali Ghei.

SHE IS GONE (HE IS GONE)

She Is Gone (He Is Gone)
You can shed tears that she is gone
Or you can smile because she has lived
You can close your eyes and pray that she will come back
Or you can open your eyes and see all that she has left
Your heart can be empty because you can't see her
Or you can be full of the love that you shared
You can turn your back on tomorrow and live yesterday
Or you can be happy for tomorrow because of yesterday
You can remember her and only that she is gone
Or you can cherish her memory and let it live on
You can cry and close your mind, be empty and turn your back
Or you can do what she would want: smile, open your eyes, love and go on.

by David Harkins

DO NOT STAND AT MY GRAVE AND WEEP

Do not stand at my grave and weep
I am not there. I do not sleep.
I am a thousand winds that blow.
I am the diamond glints on snow.
I am the sunlight on ripened grain.
I am the gentle autumn rain.
When you awaken in the morning's hush
I am the swift uplifting rush
Of quiet birds in circled flight.
I am the soft stars that shine at night.

Do not stand at my grave and cry;
I am not there. I did not die.

by Mary Elizabeth Frye

LOSS IS MORE

Loss is more than grief
More than death
More than fear
More than change.
Loss brings a new normal—but nothing's normal; it's all unknown.
Loss has physical roots, intellectual metacognition, social pain, emotional ties; it is
spiritual and visceral.
Housed in foundational places of our lives—loss leaves us unsettled, unbalanced,
provoked with anxiety.
But most difficultly, is still going on, dealing with life after loss.
No wonder loss is so hard!

by Maple Melder Crozier, 17 May 2018, my birthday, 1 week post funeral

[I CARRY YOUR HEART WITH ME(I CARRY IT IN]

i carry your heart with me (i carry it in
my heart) i am never without it (anywhere
i go you go, my dear; and whatever is done
by only me is your doing, my darling)
i fear
no fate (for you are my fate, my sweet) i want
no world (for beautiful you are my world, my true)
and it's you are whatever a moon has always meant
and whatever a sun will always sing is you

here is the deepest secret nobody knows
(here is the root of the root and the bud of the bud
and the sky of the sky of a tree called life; which grows
higher than the soul can hope or mind can hide)
and this is the wonder that's keeping the stars apart

i carry your heart (i carry it in my heart)

by e.e. cummings

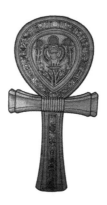

Quotes, Questions, Comments
& Signs from Beyond

"There is no grief like the grief that does not speak."
Henry Wadsworth Longfellow

At times, a short quote can be an encouragement to those grieving. Here are a few of my favourites:

What I have learned is that everyone is grieving.
Ricky Gervais, British actor

The final stage of healing is using what happens to you to help other people.
Gloria Steinem, American feminist activist and philosopher

Tears are the silent language of grief.
Voltaire, French philosopher

There is no grief like the grief that does not speak.
Henry Wadsworth Longfellow, American poet

Grief is the price we pay for love.
Queen Elizabeth II, British monarch

It takes strength to make your way through grief, to grab hold of life and let it pull you forward.
Patti Davis, daughter of President Ronald Reagan

When grief is deepest, words are fewest.
Ann Voskamp, Canadian author

No one ever told me that grief feels so much like fear.
C.S. Lewis, British novelist

The people who love you will change you.
Gramma Tala, from the Disney movie *Moana*

We all lose those we love and this is a great unifying trust amongst humans.
Shilpi Somay Gowda, Canadian Author in novel The Shape of Family

She thought nothing could ever be as bad as losing her brother.
His loss had damaged her so irreversibly that she had never found

her equilibrium again. **Every loss she suffered now hurt her more, not less.**
Shilpi Somay Gowda, Canadian Author in novel <u>The Shape of Family</u>

God has . . . set eternity in the human heart.
Ecclesiastes 3: 11, New International Version Bible

By the time we learn to live, it's already too late.
Aragon, French poet

Music is no more than the sound of our regrets put to a cadence that stirs the illusion of hope.
Andre Acuman, Italian-American author

He who is not busy being born is busy dying.
Roger McGuinn, American songwriter

An examined death is as important as an examined life.
Julia Samuel, British author and psychotherapist

Whenever you see flies or insects in a still life—a wilted petal, a black spot on the apple—the painter is giving you a secret message. He's telling you that living things don't last—it's all temporary. Death in life.
Donna Tartt, American author

Finding gratitude is not in the death. It's in the life that was lived. Balance grief with play.
David Kessler, American author and grief specialist

I'll never get out of this world alive.
Hank Williams, American singer-songwriter

If I had to choose between instant death and a slow death, I would choose the latter. An instant shatters. An instant can tear down the world. The word instant was wont to give us solace. What could you prevent from happening in an instant?
Billie Livington, Canadian author

Love is worth it. It is always worth it. In fact, it's the only thing that's worth anything.
Alan Wolfert, American author and grief specialist

Death changes everything. Time changes nothing. I still miss the sound of your voice, the wisdom in your advice, the stories of your life and just being in your presence. So, no, time changes nothing. I still miss you just as much today as I did the day you died. I just miss you.

Anonymous

Even now, as broken as you may feel, you are still so strong. There's something to be said for how you hold yourself together and keep moving, even though you feel like shattering. Don't stop. This is your healing. It doesn't have to be pretty, or graceful. You just have to keep going.

Maxwell Diawuoh, American poet

I know now what matters and it is not what I have lost. It is my memories. Wounds heal. Love lasts. We remain.

Kristen Hannah, American author

If we have been pleased with life, we should not be displeased with death, since it comes from the hand of the same master.

Michelangelo, Italian sculptor

On various public websites, forums, and blogs on social media, people discuss death and loss that they have experienced. Here are a few that were mentioned multiple times, so the sentiment bears repeating:

QUESTIONS POSED BY THOSE WHO HAVE LOST LOVED ONES:

Can somebody please tell me how I can find who I am now that he's gone? I'm just so broken.

Am I still stepmom to my late husband's kids?

Have you ever wondered how your late spouse would have handled being the one left?

Anyone else have nowhere to be this long weekend?

What happens to "friends and family"? Mine seem suddenly gone! I don't understand. They were all here when he was sick.

COMMENTS MADE BY THOSE WHO HAVE LOST LOVED ONES:

I feel like I'm living in a fog. I can occasionally see where I'm going but most of the time I'm hopelessly lost in it.

One of the most valuable gifts in life is a loyal friend.

I'm struggling with living alone. We did everything together.

I lost my husband suddenly two and a half weeks ago. No one ever told me how horrible this is.

I am scared because my future is uncertain.

I experienced the gradual "cricket chirping" get louder a week or two after my spouse passed.

You guys (others on the online grief site) are my therapy.

I realize that I have been neglecting myself. Today I will push myself.

Guilt!!!

I have been struggling. It is six months since my husband passed away. I'm exhausted, I can hardly breath. I need some peace.

Sometimes the things we can't change end up changing us.

It seems to be getting worse, not better. I'm so sad and lost without the other part of me.

I love sleep. You forget about pain, problems, stress, everything—for a while.

He has been gone four years. I felt guilty all day yesterday because I was happy with my life now. I told a friend that I wouldn't want to go back, if I had a choice. I said I was different than I was then, and happy with my life. He told me something is wrong with me, and asked how I could not want my husband back. Now I feel even more guilty.

Special days are even tougher. It's my fifty-ninth birthday and exactly five months since he passed. No "Happy birthday, Beautiful!" or big hug or kisses from the one who loved me the most.

True love never dies. His is always with me.

I am not adding this year to my age. I did not use it.

COMMENTS AND QUESTIONS THAT ARE NOT HELPFUL:

How are you doing?

Are you over it yet?

How did he die?

Wow, you have been widowed twice? Are you the black widow?

Everything happens for a reason.

Are you feeling better? (I wasn't sick; my husband passed away.)

Do you think it's easier to lose them suddenly than to illness?

Are you going to stay in your house?

Exactly what happened?

Don't you think you should hang out with singles instead of couples now?

Well, at least you had time to say goodbye.

Why and how?

Are you dating?

You just need time.

Who is your contact in case of emergency?

SIGNS FROM BEYOND

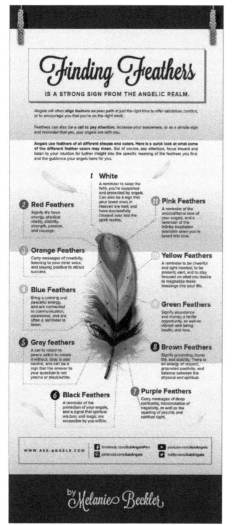

Feathers are thought to be significant signs of, or from, your deceased loved one. The different colours have meanings, and they are thought to be sent by angels to bring validation, comfort, or encouragement. I had never heard of this belief before my loss, but I certainly did notice feathers around me after I heard about this: falling from the roof, flying on the breeze, or sitting on my deck as I came home. Believe it or don't, but it was nice to think of this as an existential connection to my loved one. Below is a website that explains it:

https://www.ask-angels.com/spiritual-guidance/angel-feathers-meaning-finding-feathers/

Dimes are another item that are thought to be messages from ancestors, or deceased loved ones in a heavenly place. Seeing them means someone is trying to get your attention or guide you.

Here is one person's story about finding dimes after the loss of a loved one:

A couple of years ago, the strangest thing began happening to me. I started finding dimes all over the place. At first I didn't think much of it. But after it kept happening, I started to think it was not just a coincidence. I wasn't finding pennies, nickels, or any other coins, just dimes. It seemed like every time I turned around there was a dime, sometimes more than one.

It probably sounds silly that I would think anything of it, but it wasn't just how often I was finding them, but also the strange places they would show up. I have always felt like when something keeps happening over and over, it's a sign.

It felt like someone was leaving them for me to find. I just couldn't figure out who or why. After about the third or fourth time it happened in only two days, I started looking around thinking, okay, am I on *Candid Camera*, or what? It became a pretty regular event, so I started saving them. I wanted to see if I was actually finding as many as it seemed like I was.

THE FOLLOWING ARE POSSIBLE WAYS TO INTERPRET FINDING DIMES:

- It is a message from beyond.
- Someone or something is trying to get your attention.
- It is guidance or validation that you're on the right path.
- The dime is a reminder that you are loved and valued.
- It is a sign that positive changes are afoot.
- Ancestors, spirits, guides, or deceased loved ones want you to know they're looking out for you.
- The number 10 symbolizes a circle, so a dime might indicate coming full circle, fulfillment, unity, or the completion of a task.
- It may be a reminder to pay attention, keep watching, and keep your eyes open.

Here is a website that discusses it further:

https://exemplore.com/paranormal/Why-Do-I-Keep-Finding-Dimes-Everywhere-I-Go

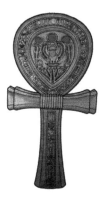

Websites & Helpful Models

"No one ever told me that grief feels so much like fear."
C.S. Lewis

These are websites I have come across in my review of literature, or during discussions with people. I do not endorse them, as many may not be right for your purposes or for your client. However, one might resonate and provide the insights and support that is needed. The information below in quotation marks is quoted from the website.

https://drjaychildrensgriefcentre.ca/
Their vision is "to build healthy and compassionate communities to support children, youth and families living with dying, death and grief." They began and exist to "meet an identified gap in psychosocial support services for children and youth who were dying and whose lives were touched by the death of parent or sibling."

http://www.griefworks.org
This organization exists "providing healing and hope to over 10,000 people - children, teens, adults, and families." They give support and "the courage to be vulnerable."

https://www.histography.co/
This is a site where you can write your life story. Note there is a fee.

https://www.nia.nih.gov/health/getting-your-affairs-order
This is a governmental site describing important documentation and end-of-life planning.

https://www.compassionatefriends.org/
This site provides a friendship group for parents who have experienced the loss of a child, as "a self-help organization offering friendship, understanding, and hope to bereaved families."

https://griefresourcenetwork.com/crisis-center/hotline/
This is a site with the most up-to-date "hotlines and online resources to help those in crisis due to the loss of a loved one."

https://www.cruse.org.uk/get-help/helpline
This website is about a helpline staffed by trained workers "who offer emotional support to anyone affected by bereavement."

https://www.bcbh.ca/
This site attempts to connect the "public to grief support services within the province of BC."

https://www.helpguide.org/articles/grief/coping-with-grief-and-loss.htm
This site has a focus on suicide and promises to be a "guide to mental health & wellness" with "healthy ways to deal with the grieving process."

https://www.centerforloss.com/
This is a well-respected organization working with issues of grief and loss, "dedicated to 'companioning' grieving people as they mourn significant transitions and losses that transform their lives." They offer education and resources.

www.hotyoungwidowsclub.com
The author states with great empathy, "We're sorry your person died. And we're here for you."

https://www.griefshare.org/
This is a faith-based site that provides online support. One participant commented that "going to GriefShare feels like having warm arms wrapped around you when you're shivering."

www.grief.com
This site is devoted to finding meaning after a loss. "The meaning is not in the death. The meaning is what we do after. The meaning is in us."

https://deathcafe.com/
This is a site providing "a Death Cafe where people drink tea, eat cake and discuss death. Our aim is to increase awareness of death to help people make the most of their (finite) lives." There are 3000 groups in thirty-four countries.

https://www.youtube.com/watch?v=khkJkR-ipfw
a funny but sincere view of grieving

https://letsreimagine.org/about
This site asks us to think about "a world in which we are all able to reflect on why we're here, prepare for a time when we won't be, and live fully right up until the end."

https://www.after.community/
A for-profit company that has "created a set of products that make it easier than ever to think through your **end-of-life wishes** with the help of your friends and family."

http://www.finalwordsproject.org/
    A linguistic analysis of people's final words before death

Strong Nations https://www.strongnations.com/ (non-academic)
    A First Nations collection of resources

www.scrapbook.com › articles › after-loss
    For-profit company that helps create scrapbooks and albums after your loss

https://whenyoulosesomeone.com/
    Resources both for those who have lost and are supporting those with loss
    And her blog: The Journey from Grief to Gratitude

**BELOW ARE SOME WEBSITES DEDICATED
TO CHILDREN'S GRIEF AND LOSS:**

https://www.kidshealth.org.nz/bereavement-reactions-children

https://www.dougy.org

https://www.youtube.com/watch?v=Nb4vXwbWd3Q

https://www.youtube.com/watch?v=Nb4vXwbWd3Q

https://www.helpguide.org/articles/caregiving/hospice-and-palliative-care.htm

MODELS
....

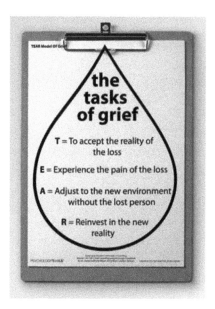

Below are two models of care for people who are grieving, developed by two prominent theorists and educators on the subject:

DR. ALAN WOLFELT

<u>Companioning</u> is an idea of providing ongoing one-on-one support to someone who has lost a loved one. A volunteer is trained and meets with a bereaved person regularly, as a companion.

<u>Tenets of Companioning the Bereaved</u>

1. Being present to another person's pain; it is not about taking away the pain.

2. Going to the wilderness of the soul with another human being; it is not about thinking you are responsible for finding the way out.

3. Honoring the spirit; it is not about focusing on the intellect.

4. Listening with the heart; it is not about analyzing with the head.

5. Bearing witness to the struggles of others; it is not about judging or directing these struggles.

6. Walking alongside; it is not about leading.

7. Discovering the gifts of sacred silence; it is not about filling up every moment with words.

8. Being still; it is not about frantic movement forward.

9. Respecting disorder and confusion; it is not about imposing order and logic.

10. Learning from others; it is not about teaching them.

11. Compassionate curiosity; it is not about expertise.

DR. DAVID KESSLER

"Finding Meaning" Theory

David Kessler has been a therapist specializing in grief and loss for several years. After he experienced the loss of a child, he reviewed his work and added the concept of meaning from loss. This book and an offered course present this material to help survivors find meaning after a loss.

The Five Areas of Grief

1. Understanding

2. Healing

3. The Mind in Grief

4. Legacy

5. Continued Connection

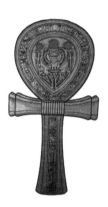

Conclusion

"I know now what matters and it is not what I have lost.
It is my memories. Wounds heal. Love lasts. We remain."

Kristen Hannah, author

CONCLUDING THOUGHTS

It has been a privilege to listen to the stories shared by these eleven people about the death of their loved ones, and to hear from those who shared personal anecdotes. The overriding sentiment from those interviewed was that they were glad to tell the story. They wanted to share and keep the memory of their loved one present, even though the loved one is a memory. Though it caused them pain, and brought tears, they wanted to tell the story.

Most of those who were interviewed had made their peace with the death, not right away, but since the loss. They had supports in place if needed, for their own emotional support, and for their families. Most were doing well, by their own report. But they didn't want to lose the memories, and felt that with time, the memories, the stories, the moments, were slipping away.

Many interviewees and anecdotal contacts said they wish they could just talk about their loved one without judgment. They felt friends and family thought, or at times said, "It's been a year; are you still talking about him?" Giving people a safe place to replay these memories is one mission of most hospice organizations. For many, I compared it to looking through a photo album or watching old home movies. It brings back a story and a smile.

Moving on is a misnomer—it should be *moving through* . . . and through . . . like dense fog or a white-out blizzard that obscures one's vision completely at first, but slowly, with time, allows movement, then some light, and then, hopefully, eventually, clear vision again.

Another universal thought from those interviewed was the desire to help others understand grief and loss, as far as they could, from their experience. They collectively said that they wished our culture would give this education to us all, especially children, that death is a part of life.

"We are forever changed by the experience of loss" (Wolfelt, 2016).

All grief and losses have guilt associated with them. It may or may not be deserved, but not understanding that guilt is what makes it so difficult to reconcile. At the right time, it's significant to venture into the messy, uncomfortable parts of the death, so guilt can be reflected upon. There may be a commonality with survivor guilt, in which those left behind feel guilty they are alive. There may be the presence of self-pity at the unfairness. But guilt is present in some form.

Sudden death versus death from a life-limiting illness both have positives and negatives. We don't usually get to choose which our loved one has. They are not to be compared, one better or worse. Those interviewed often felt the one they didn't experience would have been so much harder. Every death is difficult and has its own challenges; it isn't productive to make comparisons.

There are many resources available to make our own death process a little lighter for our loved ones. This planning does force us to confront our own mortality, which could be why many people don't engage, as these can be tough discussions. This confrontation of our own mortality becomes a realization for people who are grieving.

The cliché "There are no atheists in foxholes," was not upheld by all my interviewees. Some lost their faith through the death of their loved one. Others came to faith. There was no one accepted truth regarding afterlife and faith in it. Those with a belief in some form of afterlife felt they had an easier time coping with the parting, since they had the hope of meeting their loved one again. Discussions and exploration of some form of afterlife appeared valuable to most, as most mentioned it.

A final suggestion is that we need a wider vocabulary for discussions of death and loss. We have multiple words for love and for sex. Why not for death? Real words that objectively help us understand, rather than euphemistic offerings that allow us to skirt the issue.

MY EPILOGUE

I have started to put my own affairs in order to make it easier for my kids.

Being someone new to this forced role transition—widow, single, alone—is frightening, especially after being a wife and partner for over forty years. On a trip recently, I was asked twice if I was travelling alone. Both went on to ask why, when I didn't offer an explanation. Restaurant servers regularly ask, "Eating alone today?" I want to reply with a snarky, "Yes, everyday," but I resist. How do we rebuild belonging, finding were we fit in our society with our new identity? Our community and friends dissipate. We don't have the same connections to them.

I have also come to a startling conclusion about authenticity. When I was trained as a counsellor, we learned to suppress our natural emotional reactions, facial expressions, and body language in response to what the client was saying. In the Human Services field, we often follow that model, so as to let the client lead the encounter and to not escalate a situation. We compartmentalize our reactions, to debrief at a more appropriate time with other professionals.

It is just that unnaturalness, that lack of authenticity, that made my interviewees upset when people spoke to them about the death of their loved ones. They wanted to see the pain in the eyes of their listeners, to know the burden was shared. They wanted to know others felt the loss.

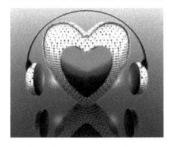

Another thought about grief is that it is not always "mindful." That is because it is not from the mind but the heart. It is a heart activity. It comes from deep in our selves. So, though we empathize with people using our minds to support them to be serene and at peace, grief makes us want to yell, rebel, cry, and breathe hard and pound on something.

That's why empathy is not enough. Listening is not enough. Those efforts are cognitive. Grief is visceral; the response needs to be visceral too. I call this listening with the heart.

LEGACY

I feel a sense of dread whenever I am embarking on a trip. Mike went on a trip and never came back. It's not a fear of my own death, but a worry for my kids. I don't want them to go through that pain again. Yet I know they will.

Pictures are precious! I buy Facebook memory books, and get so excited when someone unearths an old photo. I have joined the alumni associations of Mike's old junior high and high school, who have shared memories and photos with me. I love it when someone sends me an old picture of him!

There is my life before Mike died, and after. I had a wonderful life before I was with him, and a brilliant love story for over forty years, all before. Then he died. The rest of the *after* is still to be written . . .

The death of a loved one forces us to come to terms with our own mortality, and plan as we would for any other eventuality of life. We will all die.

This book is my small effort to support people to *really live*.

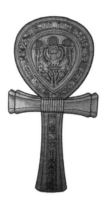

References

"By the time we learn to live, it's already too late."

Aragon, French poet

REFERENCES

Albom, M., 2002. *Tuesdays with Morrie: An Old Man, A Young Man, and Life's Greatest Lesson.* Broadway Books.

Anderson, J. (n.d.). *Jamie Anderson Quotes.* Retrieved January 2020 from https://www.goodreads.com/author/quotes/3395454.Jamie_Anderson.

Boyce, C., & Neale, P. (2006). *Conducting in-depth Interviews: A Guide for Designing and Conducting In-Depth Interviews,* Pathfinder International Tool Series. Retrieved March 2020 from https://research-methodology.net/research-methods/qualitative-research/interviews/.

Byock, I. (1988). *Dying Well.* Riverhead Books.

Cacciatore, J., & DeFrain, J. (2015). *The World of Bereavement.* Springer.

Callahan, M., & Kelley, P. (2012). *Final Gifts.* Simon & Schuster.

Coenen, C., & Pimas, M. (2020). *Creative Toolkit for working with Grief and Bereavement.* Jessica Kingsley Publishers.

Cordova, R. (2014). *Day of the Dead History.* Retrieved May 2020 from https://www.azcentral.com/story/entertainment/holidays/day-of-the-dead/2014/09/24/day-of-the-dead-history/16174911/

Cummings, E. E. (1991). *I Carry Your Heart With Me.* Retrieved September 2019 from https://www.poetryfoundation.org/poetrymagazine/poems/49493/i-carry-your-heart-with-mei-carry-it-in.

Devine, M., & Nepo, M. (2017). *It's OK That You're Not OK: Meeting Grief and Loss in a Culture That Doesn't Understand.* Sounds True, Inc., 1st Ed.

Didion, J. (2007). *The Year of Magical Thinking.* Knopf Doubleday Publishing Group, Reprint.

Dunn, B., & Leonard, K. (2004). *Through a Season of Grief.* Thomas Nelson.

Edwards, R. (2017). *Everything you need to know about Taiwan's funeral strippers.* Retrieved Dec 2020 from: https://metro.co.uk/2017/10/02/dying-around-the-world-everything-you-need-to-know-about-taiwans-funeral-strippers-6962458/.

Fink, J. (2017). *When You Lose Someone You Love.* Companion House Books.

Fisher, N. (2018). *The History of Hospice: A different kind of "care".* Retrieved February 2020 from https://www.forbes.com/sites/nicolefisher/2018/06/22/the-history-of-hospice-a-different-kind-of-health-care.

Franklin, B. (n.d.). *Phrase Finder.* Retrieved January 2021 from https://www.phrases.org.uk/meanings/death-and-taxes.html.

Freeman, C. (2015). *The Widow's Journal: Questions to Guide You Through Grief and Life Planning After the Loss of a Partner.* Create Space Independent Publishing Platform.

Gawande, A. (2017). *Being Mortal.* Picador, 1st Ed.

Gladwell, M. (2019). *Talking to Strangers.* Abacus/Hachette USA/Penguin.

Guthke, K. (1992). *Last Words.* Princeton University Press, Revised Expanded Ed.

Halifax, J. & Byock, I. (2009). *Being with Dying.* Shambhala, Reprint Ed.

Hospice of Holland (2019). *A Brief History of Hospice.* Retrieved from https://understandhospice.org/brief-history-hospice/#:~:text=The%20first%20of%20such%20hospices,as%20religious%20orders%20became%20dispersed.&text=Saunders%20showed%20pictures%20of%20patients,after%20receiving%20specialized%20hospice%20care.

James, J., Friedman, R., & Matthews, L. (2002). *When Children Grieve.* Harper Perennial, Reprint Ed.

Karst, P. (2018). *The Invisible String.* Little, Brown Books for Young Readers

Keeley, M., & Yingling, J. (2007). *Final Conversations.* Vanderwyk & Burnham, 1st Ed.

Kessler, D. (2020). *Finding Meaning: The Sixth Stage of Grief.* Scribner.

Kubler Ross, E. (2014). *On Death and Dying, 50th Anniversary Ed.* Scribner, 1st Ed.

Lewis, C. S. (2015). *A Grief Observed.* Harper One, 1st Ed.

Livingston, B. (2016). *The Crooked Heart of Mercy.* Random House Canada.

McRaven, W. (2014). *Make Your Bed*. Retrieved September 2019 from https://james-clear.com/great-speeches/make-your-bed-by-admiral-william-h-mcraven

McInerny, N. (2019). *The Hot Young Widows Club*. Simon & Schuster/TED.

Moody, R. (2015). *Life After Life*. Harper One.

Murthy, V. (2020). *Together: The Healing Power of Human Connection in a Sometimes-Lonely World*. Harper Wave.

Nuland, S. (2008). *How We Die: Reflections on Life's Final Chapter*. Paw Prints.

Parr, T. (2015). *The Goodbye Book*. Little, Brown Books for Young Readers

Pitawanakwat, K. (2015). *When My Son Died*. (Self-published.)

Pocket Guide (n.d.). *The Maori Haka: Its Meaning & History*. Retrieved Jan 2021 from https://nzpocketguide.com/the-maori-haka-its-meaning-history/

Prechtel, M. (2015). *The Smell of Rain on Dust: Grief and Praise*. North Atlantic Books.

Rappaport, H. (2012). *Magnificent Obsession*. Retrieved March 2021 from https://www.theguardian.com/books/2012/jan/20/magnificent-obsession-helen-rappaport-review.

Rasmussen, C. (2013). *Second Firsts: Live, Laugh, and Love Again*. Hay House, Inc., 1st Ed.

Rinpoche, S., Gaffney, P., & Harvey, A. (2020). *The Tibetan Book of Living and Dying*. Harper San Francisco, 1st Ed.

Salisbury, K., 2019. *Where The Tradition of Wearing Black To A Funeral Comes From*. Retrieved March 2021 from https://www.kirstysalisbury.com/blog-posts/where-the-tradition-of-wearing-black-to-a-funeral-comes-from

Samuel, J. (2018). *Grief Works*. Scribner.

Smartt, L., & Moody, R. (2017). *Words at the Threshold: What We Say as We're Nearing Death*. New World Library.

Stein, G., & Alley, R. W. (2014). *Enzo Races in the Rain!* Harper Collins.

Stein, G. (2018). *The Art of Racing in the Rain*. Harper.

Taiwan Guide (n.d.). *Taiwan Country Guide: Language, Customs, Culture, & Etiquette*. Retrieved June 2020 from https://www.commisceo-global.com/resources/country-guides/taiwan-guide.

Tartt, D., 2013. *The Goldfinch: A Novel*. Little, Brown and Company; American First edition.

Teckentrup, B. (2014). *The Memory Tree*. Orchard Books.

Thistle, J. (2019). *From the Ashes. My story of being Metis, homeless, and finding my way*. Simon & Schuster.

Thomas, A. (2007). *A Three Dog Life*. Harvest Books.

Thomas, A. (2016). *What Comes Next and How to Like It*. Scribner, Reprint.

Thomas, P., & Harker, L. (2001). *I Miss You*. B. E. S., 1st Ed.

University of the Fraser Valley, 2016. *Collective Agreement*, 2016-2019. UFV Press.

Wilhelm, H. (1988). *I'll Always Love You*. Dragonfly Books.

Wolfelt, A. (2003). *Healing a Spouse's Grieving Heart*. Companion Press.

Wolfelt, A. (2016). *When Your Soulmate Dies*. Companion Press.

COUNTRY AND CULTURE INFORMATION, RETRIEVED APRIL 2021 FROM

https://www.commisceo-global.com/resources/country-guides/taiwan-guide

https://timetravelbee.com/places/p-indonesia/facts-about-balinese-culture/

https://www.funeralwise.com/customs/samoan/

https://www.innovacareconcepts.com/en/blog/news/a-brief-history-of-hospices/

https://understandhospice.org/brief-history-hospice/

https://www.talkdeath.com/cultures-that-celebrate-death/

BIBLE VERSES, RETRIEVED JANUARY 2019 FROM

https://www.biblegateway.com/passage/?search=Proverbs+3%3A5%2C+6&version=NLT

https://www.biblegateway.com/passage/?search=2+Corinthians+1%3A4&version=NIV

https://www.biblegateway.com/passage/?search=Ecclesiastes+3&version=NIV